Clinical Management of Renal Cell Cancer

Titles of Related Interest

Smith, Middleton/*Clinical Management of Prostatic Cancer,* 1987

Soloway, Hardeman/*Clinical Management of Bladder Cancer* (to be published)

Clinical Management of Renal Cell Cancer

JAMES E. MONTIE, M.D.
Chairman, Department of Urology
Cleveland Clinic Florida
Fort Lauderdale, Florida

Associate Editors

J. EDSON PONTES, M.D.
Head, Section of Urologic Oncology
Department of Urology
Cleveland Clinic Foundation
Cleveland, Ohio

RONALD M. BUKOWSKI, M.D.
Associate Director of Clinical Research
Cleveland Clinic Cancer Center
Staff Physician
Department of Hematology and Medical Oncology
Cleveland Clinic Foundation
Cleveland, Ohio

YEAR BOOK MEDICAL PUBLISHERS, INC.
CHICAGO • LONDON • BOCA RATON • LITTLETON, MASS.

1   2   3   4   5   6   7   8   9   0   Y   R   94   93   92   91   90

Library of Congress Cataloging-in-Publication Data

Montie, James E.
    Clinical management of renal cell cancer / James E. Montie, J. Edson Pontes, Ronald M. Bukowski.
        p.   cm.
    Includes bibliographical references.
    ISBN 0-8151-5942-0
    1. Kidneys—Cancer.   I. Pontes, J. Edson.   II. Bukowski, Ronald M.
III. Title.
    [DNLM: 1. Carcinoma, Renal Cell. 2. Kidney—surgery. 3. Kidney Neoplasms—therapy.   WJ 358 M781c]
RC280.K5M66   1990   90-12187
616.99'461—dc20   CIP
DNLM/DLC
for Library of Congress

Sponsoring Editor: David K. Marshall
Associate Managing Editor, Manuscript Services: Deborah Thorp
Production Project Coordinator: Carol A. Reynolds
Proofroom Supervisor: Barbara M. Kelly

Contributors

RONALD M. BUKOWSKI, M.D.
Associate Director of Clinical Research
Cleveland Clinic Cancer Center
Staff Physician
Department of Hematology and Medical Oncology
Cleveland Clinic Foundation
Cleveland, Ohio

HOWARD S. LEVIN, M.D.
Pathologist
Cleveland Clinic Foundation
Cleveland, Ohio

JAMES E. MONTIE, M.D.
Chairman, Department of Urology
Cleveland Clinic Florida
Fort Lauderdale, Florida

ANDREW C. NOVICK, M.D.
Chairman, Department of Urology
Cleveland Clinic Foundation
Cleveland, Ohio

J. EDSON PONTES, M.D.
Head, Section of Urologic Oncology
Department of Urology
Cleveland Clinic Foundation
Cleveland, Ohio

Preface

A urologist's or medical oncologist's current perception of progress in the care of the patient with renal cell carcinoma (RCC) is often contradictory. No reliable "breakthrough" has occurred in the treatment of metastatic disease despite tantalizing prospects with biologic response modifier (BRM) therapy. A narrow viewpoint might thus imply that nothing really new is evident with this disease.

However, there truly have been remarkable changes in the diagnosis and treatment of RCC in the 10 to 15 years since the last book on this topic was published in the 1970s. Imaging of the kidney with ultrasonography, computed tomography, and magnetic resonance imaging has not only altered the way that patients are evaluated preoperatively, but has fundamentally changed the manner in which the diagnosis is even established in many cases. We are hopeful that this improved diagnostic ability will ultimately be translated into a survival benefit. There have also been major advances in the technical aspects of partial nephrectomy and inferior vena cava tumor thrombectomy, procedures rarely performed and poorly understood 15 years ago.

This book should assist the urologist, radiologist, and medical oncologist in the diagnosis and treatment of RCC. It is a review designed to allow quick, concise access to the important clinical, imaging, and pathologic differential diagnostic characteristics of RCC. This reflects a practical approach to decision-making and treatment. The present format has not been used previously and we hope it is valuable.

The recommendations for therapy are based to a large degree on experience from the Cleveland Clinic, representing one of the largest series in the world with partial nephrectomy, radical nephrectomy, and inferior vena cava tumor thrombectomy. A 15-year history of research in the BRM therapy for RCC has culminated in the trials of adoptive immunotherapy with tumor infiltrating lymphocytes and in the study of several new cytokines.

The last decade has been a time of innovation and progress in the management of RCC and we hope that *Clinical Management of Renal Cell Cancer* reflects this progress.

JAMES E. MONTIE, M.D.
J. EDSON PONTES, M.D.
RONALD M. BUKOWSKI, M.D.

Acknowledgments

Many individuals have contributed to the development of this book and we would like to thank them.

Our early mentors provided invaluable direction, guidance, and example: Ralph Straffon at the Cleveland Clinic, Willet Whitmore at Memorial Sloan-Kettering Cancer Center, Jim Pierce at Wayne State University, and Jim Hewlett at the Cleveland Clinic.

Radiology colleagues at both the Cleveland Clinic Foundation and Cleveland Clinic Florida helped with examples of specific imaging studies: Barb Risius, Mike Geisinger, and Dave Paushter at the Cleveland Clinic in Cleveland, and Maureen Sullivan and Jim Zelch at the Cleveland Clinic Florida in Ft. Lauderdale.

The photography and art departments at the Cleveland Clinic have provided timely and expert assistance.

David Marshall at Year Book Medical Publishers has been particularly patient and supportive.

Secretaries Laurie Martel and Betty White have often had the hardest job. Lorraine Caldwell has been indispensable not only in her work but also with her moral support.

JAMES E. MONTIE, M.D.
J. EDSON PONTES, M.D.
RONALD M. BUKOWSKI, M.D.

Introduction

There are several aspects of *Clinical Management of Renal Cell Cancer* that are unique and deserve emphasis. First, as far as we're aware there has not been a major text in English on renal cell cancer in approximately 15 years, and there have been rather marked changes in the diagnosis and treatment of this disease in the intervening period. Thus, the coverage of several aspects of renal cell carcinoma is fragmentary. If an individual needs to know a great deal about the imaging aspects of renal cell cancer and its differential diagnosis, he would have to refer to a radiology textbook (which wouldn't provide information on pathology or clinical situations), to a pathology textbook (which wouldn't provide radiology or clinical information), or to a general urologic oncology textbook (which often has very limited pathology and imaging correlation; when both are present they are often not in the same place). When a clinician sees a patient with a renal mass, he can review the clinical characteristics, which might give a clue to the diagnosis; review the imaging studies, which might provide additional clues; and see how the pathologic findings fit in. Before the publication of *Clinical Management of Renal Cell Cancer,* this has not been available in any other textbook. The clinician can also then proceed to the therapeutic chapters and find specific information on the surgical treatment, adjunctive measures, and specialized surgical treatment, such as partial nephrectomy or inferior vena cava tumor thrombectomy. Even very common conditions, such as incidental renal masses, are presented with very specific treatment approaches. Information is provided on the most current treatments being evaluated for metastatic disease and some of the controversies surrounding the treatments are discussed. The large number of illustrations correlating imaging and pathologic findings constitutes a unique approach.

The individual authors from the Cleveland Clinic are well established and respected individuals in the field of pathology, urology, or medical oncology, and are experts in the field of urologic oncology. The Cleveland Clinic has had one of the largest experiences in the world with RCC and the information in the book has been derived in large degree from that experience, which was obtained by direct patient care. It is our hope that the many lessons that we have learned are transmitted to the reader.

JAMES E. MONTIE, M.D.
J. EDSON PONTES, M.D.
RONALD M. BUKOWSKI, M.D.

Contents

Part I

Diagnosis

1

Epidemiology

J. Edson Pontes, M.D.

It has been estimated that approximately 19,000 cases of renal cell carcinoma (RCC) occur in the United States each year.[1] Approximately 7,000 deaths occur annually as a result of this disease.[1] Despite significant progress in the diagnosis and surgical therapy of RCC, little is known about the epidemiology of this tumor.

CAUSE

RCC is most common in patients between age 50 and 60 years. These tumors are rare in childhood, and there is a predominance of male patients to female patients of 3:1.[2] There have been only occasional studies in the cause and epidemiology of RCC. Because of the increased incidence in the male population, hormonal factors have been implicated. Experimental studies have shown that gold hamsters that are fed estrogen have developed tumors, and this animal model has been used for the study of this malignancy.[3] Chemical carcinogens have also been implicated with agents such as dimethylamine and lead acetate, which have been used to produce tumors in experimental animals.[4,5]

More recently, studies[6] of familial RCC associated with von Hippel-Lindau disease have pointed to a specific chromosomal translocation. In patients with nonfamilial RCC, we also have recently demonstrated specific nonrandom chromosomal changes involving rearrangements of chromosome 3 in 12 of 27 tumors.[7] Because all break points were clustered from p11 to p21, and two oncogenes (raf-1 and k-ras-1) have been localized in chromosome 3, it is possible that those oncogenes may be associated with the genesis of RCC. Factors responsible for the activation of such a process are presently unknown.

NATURAL HISTORY

The difficulties associated with the study of the natural history of RCC have been addressed previously by Ritchie and Chisholm.[8] The completeness of the registry of clinically presented cases is important, and the registration of un-recognized tumors will depend on the rate of autopsies for patients dying of unrelated causes. In a series reported by Hellsten et al[9] among 16,294 autopsies, 350 cases of RCC were found, 235 of which had not been known clinically. Data also have been collected in Scotland, suggesting that the incidence of RCC has been increasing in the male population as compared with a stable incidence in the female population during the same period of follow-up.[8] One of the difficulties in analyzing the incidence of unsuspected RCC found in autopsy examinations is the difference between adenoma and RCC. Controversy exists over whether the popular definition of the size of lesions less than 2 cm is valid, as some authors believe that renal adenomas are only small RCCs, since on rare occasions those tumors have been shown to be capable of metastasizing.[10, 11]

The natural history of RCC is often unpredictable. Although some data are available on the survival of patients with untreated RCC, reporting a 3- and 5-year survival of 4.4% and 2.7%, respectively, reports also are available on the development of metastatic disease 20 years after the removal of the primary and spontaneous regression of metastasis.[8, 12] This unusual biologic behavior has given rise to the speculation of the importance of the immune system in this disease and has led to current trials with biologic response modifiers.[13] Despite the curiosity that spontaneous regression has generated among investigators, this occurs infrequently and it has been reported in only about 0.3% to 0.5% of cases.[14, 15] Another unusual characteristic of this tumor is its association with paraneoplastic syndromes such as polycythemia, hypercalcemia, hepatic dysfunction, and fever of unknown origin in the absence of metastasis.[8] Despite its unusual characteristics, prognostic factors have been defined on the basis of the extent of the disease, clinical staging, and histopathologic characteristics.[16]

Staging has a distinct correlation with survival, as the presence of either distant metastasis or positive lymph nodes influences the outcome of surgery. Other investigators have looked primarily at the histologic pattern of the disease, which demonstrated that tumors with clear, granular, or oncocytic cells did much better than those containing sarcomatoid patterns.[16] The significance of renal vein involvement has been controversial and appears to relate more to the extent of the primary tumor.[17]

More recently the use of flow cytometry has been added to the histologic characteristics in an attempt to better define prognosis.[18] Although there is a relationship of aneuploidy with high grade tumors, the value of this new technology remains under investigation. In patients with metastatic disease, the natural history of this tumor has been better defined.[19] Because this tumor is resistant to most treatments available, it is easy to determine the natural history of patients with metastatic disease. In a report published by de Kernion,[19] cumulative survival of patients with metastasis was 43% at 1 year, 26% at 2 years, and 13% at 5 years. Survival was better for patients with lung metastasis only than for those with local recurrence. In that series excision of metastatic foci improved survival up to 5 years in contrast to our own experience, which reveals only improvement of survival at 2 years but no advantage at 5 years.[20] Palliative nephrectomy did not appear to influence survival in the de Kernion series, which was similar to other previous reports.[19–21]

In summary, there are no known specific causes, such as environmental factors, responsible for the development of RCC. Nonfamilial genetic markers are now being identified and in the future could shed some light on the cause of this disease.

Although the natural history of RCC is occasionally unpredictable, patients with metastatic disease have a dismal prognosis.

REFERENCES

1. Silverberg, E: Cancer statistics. *CA* 1983; 33:9.
2. Bennington JL: Cancer of the kidney—etiology, epidemiology, and pathology. *Cancer* 1973; 32:1017.
3. Horning ES, Whittick JW: Histogenesis of stilboestrol-induced renal tumors in golden male hamster. *Br J Cancer* 1954; 8:451.
4. Ireton HJC, McGiven AR, Davies DJ: Renal mesenchymal tumors induced in rats by dimethylnitrosamine: Light and electron-microscope studies. *J Pathol* 1972; 108:181.
5. Boyland E, Dukes CE, Grover PL, et al: The induction of renal tumors by feeding lead acetate to rats. *Br J Cancer* 1962; 16:283.
6. Wang N, Perkins KL: Involvement of band 3p 14 in t (3;8) hereditary renal carcinoma. *Cancer Genet Cytogenet* 1984; 11:479.
7. Yoshida M, Dhyashiki H, Ochi H, et al: Cytogenetic studies of tumor tissue from patients with nonfamilial renal cell carcinoma. *Cancer Res* 1986; 46:2139.
8. Ritchie AWS, Chisholm GD: The natural history of renal carcinoma. *Semin Oncol* 1983; 10:390.
9. Hellsten S, Berge T, Wehlin I: Unrecognized renal cell carcinoma. Clinical and diagnostic aspects. *Scand J Urol Nephrol* 1981; 8:269.
10. Hellsten S, Berge T, Wehlin L: Unrecognized renal cell carcinoma. Clinical and pathological aspects. *Scand J Urol Nephrol* 1981; 8:273.
11. Bell ET: *Renal diseases.* Philadelphia, Lea & Febiger, 1950, pp 428.
12. Tandon PL, Kuman M, Hafeez MA: Metastasis from renal cell carcinoma 20 years after nephrectomy. A case report. *Br J Urol* 1963; 35:30.
13. Pontes JE: Immunotherapy in the treatment of metastatic renal adenocarcinoma, in de Kernion J, Pavone-Macaluso M (eds): *Tumors of the Kidney.* Philadelphia, Williams & Wilkins Inc, 1986, p 274.
14. Bloom HJG: Proceedings: Hormone-induced and spontaneous regression of metastatic renal cancer. *Cancer* 1973; 32:1066.
15. de Kernion JB, Berry D: The diagnosis and treatment of renal cell carcinoma. *Cancer [Suppl]* 1980; 45:1947.
16. Boxer RJ, Waismian J, Lieber MM, et al: Renal carcinoma: Computer analysis of 96 patients treated by nephrectomy. *J Urol* 1979; 122:598.

17. Rafla S: Renal cell carcinoma. Natural history and results of treatment. *Cancer* 1970; 25:26.

18. Hofstadter F, Jakse G, Rauschmeier H, et al: The value of DNA cytophotometry for the prognostic evaluation of renal adenocarcinoma, in de Kernion J, Pavone-Maca-luso M (eds): *Tumors of the Kidney.* Philadelphia, Williams & Wilkins Inc., 1986, p 34.

19. de Kernion JB, Ramming KP, Smith RB: The natural history of metastatic renal cell carcinoma: A computer analysis. *J Urol* 1978; 120:148.

20. Pontes JE, Huben R, Novick A, et al: Salvage surgery for renal cell carcinoma. *Semin Oncol* 1989, in press.

21. Johnson DE, Kaesler KE, Samuels ML: Is nephrectomy justified in patients with metastatic renal cell carcinoma? *J Urol* 1975; 114:27.

2

Detection and Diagnosis of Renal Cell Carcinoma

James E. Montie, M.D.

Howard S. Levin, M.D.

SIGNS AND SYMPTOMS

The detection of renal cell carcinoma (RCC) has evolved significantly in the last 50 years. RCC has been characterized by an associated high frequency of unusual symptoms. The tumor was compared previously with tuberculosis and syphilis as the "great imitators" because of challenges posed to establish the diagnosis. Unless the classic triad of RCC of pain, mass, and hematuria was evident, the cancer was often unrecognized. In the 1960s, the term *internist's tumor* was coined, stressing the systemic symptoms seen with RCC.[1]

Now the systemic symptoms of RCC still are seen, but the diagnostic dilemma is less difficult because of vastly improved abdominal imaging studies. An individual with any symptoms or signs that might be caused by a neoplasm generally receives an abdominal computed tomographic (CT) scan or ultrasonography early in the evaluation; these studies are effective in identifying a mass lesion in the kidney, which might be RCC. Delays in the diagnosis, frequently 6 to 12 months in the past, are seen less often.

It is valuable to appreciate the signs and symptoms that can be caused by RCC (Table 2–1). Not only can they be seen at the time of diagnosis but they may become evident later in the course of the disease; prompt recognition can prevent or ameliorate severe consequences. Table 2–1 will also serve as an outline for the review of the various signs and symptoms encountered in caring for the patient with RCC.

TABLE 2–1.
Signs and Symptoms Related to RCC

Genitourinary
  Pain
  Mass
  Hematuria
  Varicocele
  Vaginal or penile metastases
Endocrinologic
  Hypercalcemia
  Adrenocorticotropic hormone
  Human chorionic gonadotropin
  Enteroglucagon
  Insulin-like
  Prolactin
  Thyroid metastases
Abdominal
  Nonspecific gastrointestinal complaints
  Acute abdomen caused by spontaneous hemorrhage
  Stauffer's syndrome
  Elevated alkaline phosphatase level
  Budd-Chiari syndrome
Hematologic
  Anemia
  Erythrocytosis
  Elevated haptoglobin
  Leukemoid reaction
Pulmonary and cardiovascular
  Metastases
  Hypertension
  High output state
  Atrial extension
Neurologic
  Metastases
  Polyneuritis
Musculoskeletal
General
  Fever
  Amyloidosis

Genitourinary Symptoms

Hematuria, either gross or microscopic, is the most common symptom or sign of RCC. Approximately 60% of patients will have hematuria, usually gross and painless unless there is colic secondary to obstruction of the upper tract from a clot.[2] Prolonged periods can occur between episodes of bleeding. The degree of hematuria can vary from microscopic only to heavy bleeding with clot retention in the bladder.

It is important to note that 30% to 40% of patients with RCC will not have

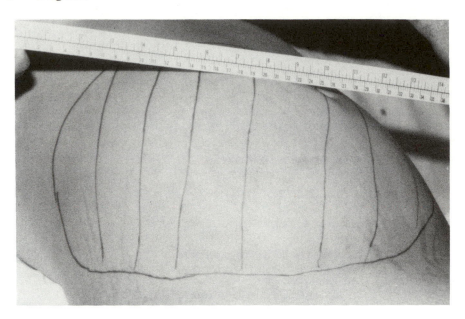

FIG 2–1.
Patient with 35 cm palpable abdominal mass secondary to renal carcinoma. The patient's only complaints were a vague discomfort in the abdomen and a sensation that her clothes did not fit well recently.

any hematuria. Thus the presence of a normal urinalysis does not eliminate the possibility that RCC is present.

RCC can occasionally become large (15 to 20 cm) in the absence of symptoms due to the retroperitoneal location of the kidney (Fig 2–1). A palpable upper abdominal mass can easily be confused with the liver or the spleen. Depending on the size and growth pattern of the mass, pain may become evident from distortion and/or obstruction of the collecting system or pressure on the retroperitoneal soft tissue or intraabdominal structures.

The triad of pain, mass, and gross hematuria is now seen only in approximately 10% of patients with RCC and generally indicates a more locally advanced lesion.

A frequently mentioned but uncommonly seen sign is an acute left varicocele. This is caused by obstruction of the left spermatic vein by tumor thrombus in the renal vein or by marked increased flow in the spermatic vein because of intrarenal arteriovenous shunting into the renal vein. In contradistinction to the typical varicocele due to incompetent valves in the spermatic vein, the varicocele seen with RCC does not collapse when the patient is recumbent.

Metastases to the lower genitourinary tract are not uncommon in both men and women with RCC.[3] These metastases are seen as a mass in the vagina, penis, testis, or epididymis and conceivably are related to retrograde flow of malignant cells into the ovarian or spermatic vein.

Endocrinologic Symptoms

RCC is recognized as a malignancy with potential for ectopic hormone production. Hypercalcemia is the most common manifestation. A patient can have lethargy, mental deterioration, and azotemia secondary to unrecognized, severe hypercalcemia. It has been estimated that 10% to 12% of patients with RCC will have hypercalcemia.[4] Patients with hypercalcemia frequently have minimal or no bone metastases, and a humoral substance produced by the tumor has been implicated as the cause. The first described case of humoral hypercalcemia was a patient with RCC reported by Albright in 1941.[5] It was postulated that a parathyroid hormonelike substance was secreted by the tumor; recently the likely responsible peptide has been isolated, purified, and the amino acid sequence mapped.[5] Prostaglandins also have been implicated in contributing to the hypercalcemia, and indomethacin has been used successfully on occasion to reduce the serum calcium.[6] The metabolic interactions responsible for hypercalcemia are likely to be quite complex, and osteoclast-mediated bone resorption has been postulated as the mechanism.[7]

Recognition of the hypercalcemia is extremely important because it can be life-threatening and needs to be aggressively treated with the administration of intravenous saline solution, a brisk diuresis, steroids, mithramycin, indomethacin, or reduction in the mass of the primary tumor or metastases with surgery, radiation therapy, or biologic response modifier (BRM) therapy (Chapter 7).

Other hormonal excesses associated with or produced by RCC are well documented. Examples of these substances produced with resultant clinical manifestations include adrenocorticotrophic hormone (ACTH), human chorionic gonadotropin (HCG), enteroglucagon, prolactin, insulinlike substance, and prostaglandin A.[8, 9] It is noteworthy that RCC is one of the most frequent sources of metastases to the thyroid and metastases should not be perceived as a rare event in an individual with RCC.

Abdominal Complaints

The retroperitoneal location of the kidney and the large size attained by RCC frequently lead to nonspecific gastrointestinal complaints. The pain may be perceived as more abdominal rather than flank; nausea, weight loss, and easy satiety may be prominent. Acute abdominal pain can result from a spontaneous hemorrhage from an RCC leading to a perinephric hematoma (Fig 2–2).[10] Abdominal CT has vastly simplified the evaluation of patients with these complaints.

A fascinating manifestation of RCC has been termed "*Stauffer's syndrome.*" The syndrome was described in 1961 as being characterized by reversible hepatic dysfunction in RCC patients in the absence of liver metastases; it is seen in approximately 15% of patients.[2, 11] The classic picture includes abnormalities in at least three of the five measures of hepatic function: serum alkaline phosphatase, prothrombin time, sulfobromophthalein retention, bilirubin, and α_2-globulin.[12] More recently, α-glutamyl transpeptidase and protein electrophoresis studies have been added.[11]

The cause is not presently defined but may well be secondary to endogenous production of some type of BRM. The syndrome is frequently associated with fever (47%), anemia (67%), elevated erythrocyte sedimentation rate (73%), malaise, and weight loss (47%).[11] The failure of the toxic abnormalities to normalize after nephrectomy is generally indicative of metastatic disease and is associated with a shorter survival. The presence of this syndrome is not a documented adverse factor in prognosis.

Isolated elevation of the alkaline phosphatase in the absence of hepatic metastases also has been reported.[2] Symptoms secondary to metastases to the pancreas, gallbladder, jejunum, and stomach have been described as initial complaints.

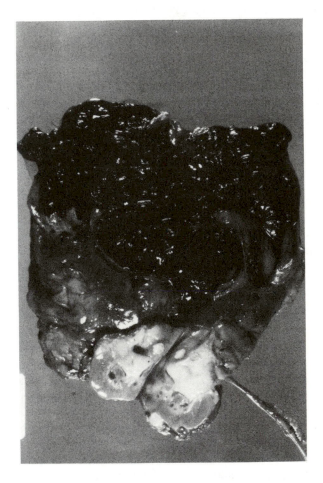

FIG 2–2.
Photograph of gross specimen of nephrectomy for small RCC associated with large spontaneous perirenal hematoma. The patient had acute abdominal pain and had an operation for a suspected incarcerated inguinal hernia. A retroperitoneal mass was then identified at the time of operation.

Rarely, RCC associated with a tumor thrombus in the intrahepatic inferior vena cava (IVC) can obstruct the hepatic veins causing an acute Budd-Chiari syndrome.

Hematologic Symptoms

Probably the most common systemic manifestation of RCC is anemia, which is generally not caused by hematuria. The anemia is noted in 20% to 30% of patients, is associated with a low serum iron and low total iron-binding capacity, and resolves after nephrectomy.[13] Loughlin et al[13] have suggested that the anemia, in at least some patients, is due to an increase in serum lactoferrin, which mediates sequestration of iron into the reticuloendothelial system. In a series of 45 patients with RCC and an IVC tumor thrombus at the Cleveland Clinic, 60% had anemia. In patients with metastases, up to 72% have anemia.[14]

Haptoglobinemia also has been reported, often associated with anemia. Leukocytosis, a leukemoid reaction, and thrombocytosis also have been described.[14]

Erythrocytosis associated with RCC has been noted but is an infrequent finding (1% to 5% of cases) and generally is mild.[14, 15] Mild elevations of plasma erythropoietin, measured with a bioassay, have been described in patients with RCC. Documentation of production by an RCC cell line of an ectopic stimulating factor, distinct from human erythropoietin, has been described by Sytkowski et al[16] in 1984.

Pulmonary and Cardiovascular Symptoms

Symptoms caused by pulmonary metastases are extremely common in RCC. Because the lung is the most frequent site of metastases and 30% to 40% of all patients with RCC have metastatic disease, recognition and management of pulmonary metastases are important. Endobronchial metastases are well described and are associated with hemoptysis and bronchial obstruction. Mediastinal lymph node and pleural metastases are frequent.[17] Differentiation between a primary renal or lung tumor can be difficult histologically and clinically.[18]

High output cardiac failure manifested by congestive heart failure, hypertension, and an abdominal bruit have been noted as resulting from massive arteriovenous shunting within the RCC.[2] A mass lesion from the tumor thrombus in the IVC extending to the right atrium or beyond can cause congestive heart failure, arrhythmias, or valvular dysfunction by prolapse through the tricuspid valve (see Figure 5–20).[19]

Hypertension may be more common in patients with RCC than in the general population.[20] Potential explanations are increased renin production by the tumor (probably rare), compression of normal parenchyma, intrarenal arteriovenous shunting with ischemia, or a high output state.

Complete obstruction of the IVC by tumor thrombus can occasionally cause peripheral edema, deep venous thrombosis, or dilated superficial veins from

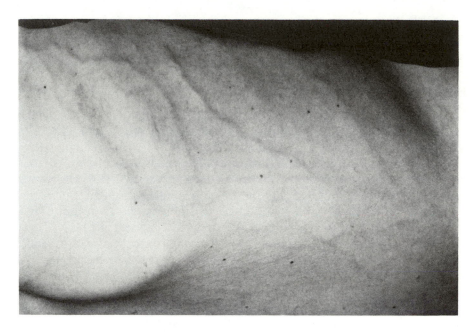

FIG 2–3.
Venous collateral circulation in the abdominal wall in a patient who has complete obstruction of the IVC as a result of RCC tumor thrombus. The patient had no peripheral edema.

marked collateral circulation (Figs 2–3 and 2–4). Benign and malignant pulmonary emboli have been seen.

Neurologic Symptoms

Most neurologic manifestations result from intracranial and vertebral body metastases.[21] Intracranial lesions are hypervascular and may need resection for significant palliation or to establish a diagnosis. Approximately half of the lesions are single, but central nervous system metastases are usually seen in conjunction with other systemic metastases. Spinal cord compression secondary to involvement and destruction of vertebral bodies is not uncommon and is a difficult problem to manage. Aggressive vertebral body resection has been advised in view of poor results with traditional treatment.[22] The pathologic diagnosis of a central nervous system metastases can be difficult because of confusion between hemangioblastoma and RCC, especially in patients with von Hippel-Lindau disease.[23]

Musculoskeletal Symptoms

Most RCC bone metastases are lytic, painful, vascular, and commonly associated with pathologic fractures. An orthopedic surgeon called on to repair a pathologic fracture from an unknown primary site may encounter extreme hemorrhage, suggesting RCC as the primary tumor. Shoulder girdle, long bones, and pelvis are common sites of metastases.[23, 24]

Systemic Symptoms

Fever secondary to RCC was described over 100 years ago. The incidence is estimated at 10%; no confirmed cause has been defined. A causal relationship to endogenous pyrogen, another BRM, or a growth factor is likely.[2]

Systemic amyloidosis has been reported previously often in association with RCC, even with prevalence up to 15% of cases.[25] A personal impression is that it is much less common than previously quoted. Clinically it may be associated with nephrotic syndrome, renal failure, and multiple organ involvement by the amyloid. Prognosis is poor.

In summary, RCC is a fascinating tumor because of its varied presentations and multiple associated manifestations. Familiarity with the range of signs and symptoms can allow earlier diagnosis of the primary lesion or of metastases,

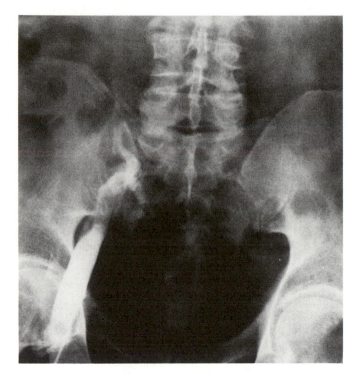

FIG 2–4.
Right femoral venogram in the same patient as in Fig 2–3 demonstrates complete occlusion of common iliac vein. The thrombus that propagated down into the iliac veins was benign but densely fibrotic and could not be removed surgically.

often minimizing morbidity. RCC can metastasize anywhere and symptoms secondary to these metastases can be the initial complaint. One should not be surprised with metastases to the prostate, retina, uvula, sinuses, etc., and any bizarre symptoms may be from the cancer.

STAGING

Staging of RCC has evolved over decades; unfortunately, confusion over the optimal approach also has increased. The dilemma is a fundamental one: does examination of more variables improve the ability to predict prognosis enough to justify the increased complexity? For example, is it valuable to identify and analyze separately patients with renal vein involvement alone versus patients with multiple levels of IVC extension, with or without perinephric fat invasion? A realistic answer is that not enough is known with certainty; efforts to accumulate data to provide meaningful guidelines are proceeding slowly.

In 1943, McDonald and Priestly[26] observed that gross tumor invasion of the renal vein had an adverse impact on survival comparable to that seen in patients with lymph node metastases. In 1958 Flocks and Kadesky[27] examined the University of Iowa experience and proposed four relatively straightforward stages.

Stage I: Limited to renal capsule.
Stage II: Invasion of renal pedicle and/or renal fat.
Stage III: Lymph node involvement.
Stage IV: Distant metastases demonstrable.

In 1963 Robson[28] reviewed a sizable experience from Toronto General Hospital and examined survival based on the presence of metastases, gross invasion of adjacent organs or renal vein, and spread to regional lymph nodes. In 1969 Robson et al[29] updated Robson's experience and then modified the staging system that ultimately became widely accepted in one form or another. The following is the staging system recommended by Robson initially:

> Stage I: Confined to kidneys.
>
> Stage II: Perirenal fat involvement but confined to Gerota's
>   fascia.
>
> Stage III:
>   *A. Gross right ventricular or IVC involvement.*
>   *B. Lymphatic involvement.*
>   *C. Vascular and lymphatic involvement.*
>
> Stage IV:
>   *A. Adjacent organs other than adrenal involvement.*
>   *B. Distant metastases.*

Thus Robson included all the variables that even now are believed to be valuable, but unfortunately, the grouping of these may not have been ideal. The analysis of survival data was done by stage without breaking out the subgroups.

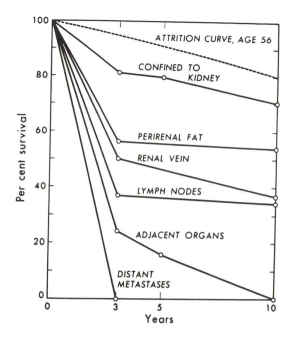

FIG 2–5.
Graph of patient survival from Robson's classic article in 1969 on the results of radical nephrectomy based on stage of the cancer. (From Robson CJ, Churchill BM, Anderson W: *J Urol* 1969; 101:297–301. Used by permission.)

If, for example, there was a difference in survival between stage III-A (positive renal vein) and stage III-B (positive lymph nodes), it would not have been observed. In a classic review in 1970 Skinner et al[30] examined the impact of these subgroups and found that the survival of stage III-A (renal vein only) was closer to stage II (perinephric fat) than to stage III-B (positive lymph nodes). Nevertheless, most subsequent reports provided data based only on the broader Robson stage I to IV classification without any breakdown within the stages. This is unfortunate because stage III really contains patients with vastly different prognoses.

Another frequently overlooked critique of the Robson system is that the conclusions were based on an extremely small number of patients. Figure 2–5 is the widely quoted graph used in Robson's article.[29] A close examination of the data indicates 5-year survival rates for stages II (invasion of perinephric fat) and III-A (invasion of renal vein) are quite close and certainly not statistically significantly different. At 10 years the difference between the curves is more striking, but the survival for perinephric fat invasion is based on only six patients, and the survival rates for renal vein invasion and positive lymph nodes are based on a total of only 13 patients. On the basis of this analysis, however, renal vein invasion was included in stage III along with invasion of lymph nodes rather than in stage II with invasion of perinephric fat. This arguable judgment has been reproduced in textbooks ever since.

TABLE 2–2.
Current American Joint Committee on Cancer Recommendations for Staging

Primary tumor (T)
  TX Primary tumor cannot be assessed
  T_0 No evidence of primary tumor
  T_1 Tumor ≤2.5 cm in greatest dimension limited to kidney
  T_2 Tumor >2.5 cm in greatest dimension limited to kidney
  T_3 Tumor extends into major veins or invades adrenal gland or perinephric tissues but not
        beyond Gerota's fascia
    T_{3a} Tumor invades adrenal gland or perinephric tissues but not beyond Gerota's fascia
    T_{3b} Tumor grossly extends into renal vein(s) or vena cava
  T_4 Tumor invades beyond Gerota's fascia
Regional lymph nodes (N)
  NX Regional lymph nodes cannot be assessed
  N_0 No regional lymph node metastasis
  N_1 Metastasis in a single lymph node, ≤2 cm in greatest dimension
  N_2 Metastasis in a single lymph node, >2 cm but not >5 cm in greatest dimension, or
        multiple lymph nodes, none >5 cm in greatest dimension
  N_3 Metastasis in a lymph node >5 cm in greatest dimension
Distant metastasis (M)
  MX Presence of distant metastasis cannot be assessed
  M_0 No distant metastasis
  M_1 Distant metastasis
Stage Grouping

Stage I:	T_1	N_0	M_0
Stage II:	T_2	N_0	M_0
Stage III:	T_1	N_1	M_0
	T_2	N_1	M_0
	T_{3a}	N_0,N_1	M_0
	T_{3b}	N_0,N_1	M_0
Stage IV:	T_4	Any N	M_0
	Any T	N_2,N_3	M_0
	Any T	Any N	M_1

The tumor, nodes, metastases (TNM) system was introduced in the United States in 1977 by the American Joint Committee on Cancer. The third edition, published in 1987, was a result of collaboration by National TNM committees from the United States, Great Britian, Canada, France, Germany, Italy, and Japan.[31] Criteria for classification identical to those proposed by the International Union Against Cancer were adopted. The attempt at promulgation of a single, simplified, worldwide system is to be applauded and supported. Table 2–2 lists the current American Joint Committee on Cancer recommendations for staging with proposed stage grouping based on similar prognoses.

Unfortunately, the changes in the second and third edition aimed at simplification can be criticized. The most noteworthy is the elimination of a separate category, T_{3c}, for IVC tumor thrombus extension; thus the present system includes both right ventricular and IVC involvement into T_{3b}. Although studies have suggested an adverse impact on survival based on increasing amounts of IVC involvement, unequivocal evidence is lacking; however, it is difficult to believe that a patient with an IVC thrombus extension into the heart has the same prognosis as someone with an isolated renal vein involvement (see Chapter 5).[32, 33] Thus for the purposes of this section we have maintained the T_{3c} category from the 1983 classification (Fig 2–6).

In 1983 an analysis of 246 patients from Cleveland Clinic Foundation was

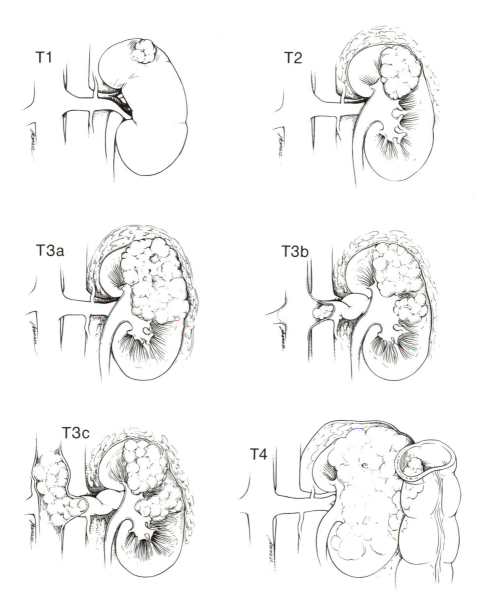

FIG 2–6.
T staging of RCC based on the American Joint Committee on Cancer criteria from 1983 and 1987.

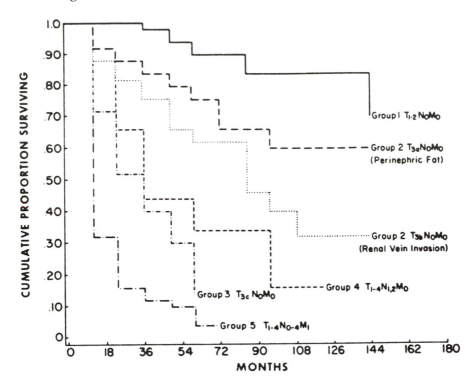

FIG 2–7.
Actuarial disease-free survival of patients relative to stage with TNM system. (From Siminovitch JPM, Montie JE, Straffon RA: *J Urol* 1983; 130:20–23. Used by permission.)

done in which multiple prognostic indicators were examined with the original TNM system.[32] Additional variables such as capsule, renal pelvic, or microscopic renal vascular invasion were examined and found to be insignificant factors. This and other studies[33, 34] validate the usefulness of the TNM system (Fig 2–7). The stage grouping as described in Figure 2–8 separated patients into groups with a statistically significant difference in prognosis for survival.[32]

The use of the TNM system should be strongly encouraged. The increased complexity in reporting the data is justified by a more accurate stratification of patients, potential for a more precise comparison between different series from several institutions, and a better prediction of the prognosis.

CLINICAL AND PATHOLOGIC FEATURES

General Imaging Aspects

Advances in imaging technology in the last 10 to 15 years have dramatically changed the process of detection of RCC. Twenty to 30 years ago an extremely common operation by a urologist was an "exploration" of a renal cyst to rule out RCC. This is an uncommon procedure today because in 95% or more of the cases the benign or malignant character of a mass can be established with certainty before surgery. Also, the difficult diagnostic dilemmas of RCC previously encountered in patients with unexplained fever, anemia, gastrointestinal complaints, etc., are resolved with the abdominal CT, which is obtained in the evaluation of unexplained abdominal complaints or in the search for occult malignancy. The clinician does not have to consciously ask "could this patient have an RCC" and then get an intravenous pyelogram (IVP), as was the course of events earlier in this century. Now the diagnosis can be made without specifically including RCC in the differential at the time of the workup.

The downside of these improvements in imaging is the potential to over use them by obtaining multiple studies in the same patient with little additional information gained. An intravenous (IV) urogram, ultrasonography, CT scan, angiography, inferior venacavography, and magnetic resonance imaging are not all necessary in each patient, and clinical judgment must be exercised. Algorithms have been developed to guide a clinician through a logical sequence of studies to establish a diagnosis.[35-37] A modification of these approaches reflecting the general philosophy is presented in Figure 2–9. These guidelines are that large or confusing lesions will need more information to sort out the diagnosis or planned therapy. The lesson to be learned in the evaluation of the renal mass lesion is to proceed with the workup until enough data are available to make a certain diagnosis; one should not stop when the lesion is regarded as "probably benign." This may require one study or it may require five studies, including surgery.

The central abnormality on any imaging study indicative of an RCC is "mass lesion" as opposed to a "filling defect" or obstruction seen typically with an

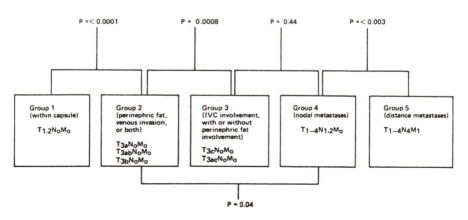

FIG 2–8.
Stage grouping to allow prediction of prognosis based on TNM staging. (From Siminovitch JPM, Montie JE, Straffon RA: *J Urol* 1983; 130:20–23. Used by permission.)

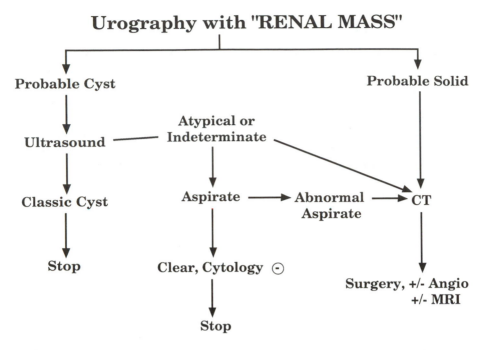

FIG 2–9.
Algorithm of guidelines for evaluation of renal mass identified on IV urogram.

epithelial cancer of the renal pelvis. Once a mass is identified, the next goal is to separate the benign cyst from the rest of the benign or malignant renal tumors or conditions. Even if one excludes the typical simple cyst, the nature of a renal mass can be determined with imaging studies in probably at least 90% of cases. In some situations biopsy or resection will be the only way to establish a firm diagnosis. The format of this section is to first discuss imaging techniques available and their general indications. Then specific radiographic and pathologic characteristics of RCC and its differential diagnoses are presented.

Intravenous Urography

Historically the urogram has been the prime study ultimately leading to the diagnosis of RCC. Currently it is probably still the most common first imaging study in the evaluation of urologic symptoms, although ultrasonography is used more frequently.

The plain film of the abdomen before injection of contrast material may provide extremely valuable information relative to the presence or character of the abdominal mass (solid, cystic, or fat), the presence of calcification within the mass, and other extra urologic findings such as displaced bowel, bone lesions, or lung nodules.[38]

Impaired renal function can be evident on the urogram suggesting renal vein obstruction. Routine tomography can ensure normal renal outlines and has been proved valuable; occasionally a mass projecting directly anteriorly or posteriorly off the surface of the kidney will not be detected (Figure 2–10).

The appearance of the mass on the urogram may give clues helpful in directing the next step. The most common mass detected in the kidney will be a renal cyst. Five percent to 15% of all patients having a urogram will have a renal cyst with a higher frequency seen with increasing age.[39, 40] Typical characteristics include a lucent appearance compared with the rest of the nephrogram, a thin, smooth wall less than 2 mm, and a "claw" or "beak" sign caused by a small amount of normal parenchyma compressed around the edge of the cyst. If these findings are present, the next reasonable step is an ultrasound examination. If this is also typical for a simple cyst, aspiration is probably not needed, and the diagnosis can be established with a 98% accuracy.[38] If any aspects of the urogram or ultrasound examination are atypical or indeterminate, aspiration of the mass or an abdominal CT scan should be done. If the appearance on the urogram suggests a lesion other than a simple cyst, we generally proceed directly to a CT scan because more overall information is obtained from this single study.

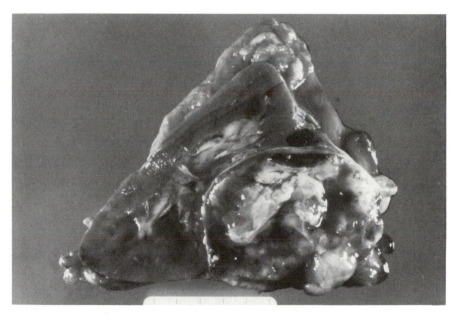

FIG 2–10.
Relatively large RCC projecting off anterior surface of kidney in a patient who had an intravenous pyelogram that was interpreted as normal. A mass projecting anteriorly or posteriorly that does not distort the collecting system can be difficult to identify on IV urography.

TABLE 2–3.
Indications for Renal CT*

1. Patients with urogram results suspicious for renal neoplasm.
2. Patients with normal urograms but suspicious signs and/or symptoms (e.g., hematuria).
3. Patients with paraneoplastic syndromes.
4. Patients with unknown primary tumors.
5. Patients with syndromes associated with renal neoplasia (e.g., von Hippel-Lindau disease), acquired renal cystic disease of dialysis.
6. Patients with previous renal cancer therapy.
7. Patients with renal scarring, focal hypertrophy, xanthogranulomatous pyelonephritis, ectopia, and fusion anomalies.

*From McClennan BL: Semin Urol 1985; III:111–131. Used by permission.

Ultrasonography

Ultrasonography represents an increasingly attractive imaging modality in urology; one of the earliest applications for this study was a mass lesion in the kidney. Lesions greater than 2 to 3 cm can be defined. The ultrasound characteristics of a simple cyst are based on the interaction of the ultrasonic waves with the low viscosity and low protein fluid in the cyst. The characteristics are the absence of an interior reflecting interface ("echo-free"), acoustic enhancement by the fluid collection, and refractive shadows adjacent to the area of acoustic enhancement.[38] The ultrasound findings indicative of a cyst are evidence of a homogeneous fluid with smooth walls, no internal septations, and a sharp demarcation from the renal parenchyma.[38]

Equipment now utilized provides a static gray scale and a real-time B-mode ultrasonoscope with either a 3.5 or 5.0 MHz transducer.[41] Patients are usually in the supine and oblique positions during the study. The quality of data depends greatly on the equipment and on the skill of the technician and/or radiologist or urologist.

Approximately 60% of patients with a cyst have a solitary, unilateral lesion, and 33% of these lesions will progress in size or number.[41] For lesions that are not absolutely typical simple cysts, aspiration of the fluid in the cyst is valuable. Clear fluid with negative results on cytology, occasionally combined with cystography confirming a smooth wall, is reliable information to rule out a malignancy. Rare exceptions have been identified. A noteworthy exception is the patient with von Hippel-Lindau disease in whom many of the cysts may have clear fluid but still harbor incipient RCC in the wall.

Computed Tomography

CT is probably the best single test to find the most information relative to mass lesions in the kidney. Indications for CT have been outlined by McClennan (Table 2–3).

Typically, scan slices are obtained at 1.0 cm intervals with a slice thickness of 1.0 cm. Scans are obtained before and after the injection of IV contrast material. Refinements in the rate, amount, and route of injection of the contrast material have been recommended in an effort to better outline the renal vessels and IVC. This has been termed "dynamic imaging."[36] Injection of IV contrast material allows an evaluation of the degree of "enhancement" of the renal mass. Renal cancers classically are less dense than the normal parenchyma before the administration of contrast material. After contrast material is given the tumor is enhanced less than the normal kidney, although if a bolus injection is given with early scanning, the neovascularity in the tumor can provide an increase in enhancement. The preferred technique by the radiologist performing the study must be appreciated.

McClennan[36] outlined the CT features of neoplasia. The indeterminate lesion should be treated as such and usually resected with either a partial or total nephrectomy as needed.

The ability of CT to stage RCC is covered under the individual characteristics used in staging. Historically, at the Cleveland Clinic we have relied more on CT than on ultrasound for diagnosis and staging. Occasionally both are needed, but we believe that CT provides more overall information. Frohmuller et al.[42] compared the urogram, ultrasonography, CT, and angiography in staging RCC and found comparable accuracy with ultrasonography (78%) and CT (72%); the urogram (59%) and angiography (57%) were less effective. In differentiating the important T_3 lesions, however, ultrasonography was accurate in 47%, but CT was accurate in 66%.

Angiography

The neovascularity of RCC with marked arteriovenous shunting, puddling, and hypervascularity is so typical for RCC that the diagnosis can often be firmly established on this basis alone. Small arterial aneurysms, parasitized capsular vessels, and large draining veins can be seen. The absence of these typical findings, however, does not rule out RCC because some necrotic or papillary lesions can be hypovascular, and small tumors can be missed entirely.

Angiography is valuable in the treatment plan of RCC, although it is used less often than it was before the era of CT. Removal of a large RCC, with or

TABLE 2–4.
CT Features of Renal Neoplasia*

   I. Mass with attenuation similar to or less than renal parenchyma.
  II. Poor definition from parenchyma.
     A. Pseudocapsule.
 III. Contrast enhancement, marked or transient.
 IV. Calcification.
     A. Central.
     B. Peripheral.
  V. Secondary signs.
     A. Lymph nodes.
     B. Venous invasion.
     C. Metastases.

*From McClennan BL: *Semin Urol* 1985; III:111–131. Used by permission.

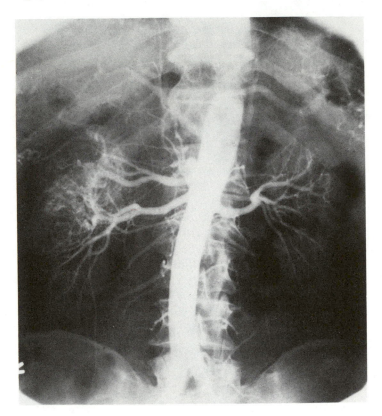

FIG 2–11.
Aortogram in patient with right RCC demonstrates two main renal arteries to the right kidney. Preoperative identification of multiple renal arteries is valuable information for the surgeon.

without renal vein or IVC involvement, can be a difficult operation, and preoperative knowledge of the arterial anatomy is valuable (Fig 2–11).

Kam et al[43] have proposed the following indications for angiography: (1) lesion is intrarenal without disruption of renal contour, (2) suspicion of a vascular abnormality, (3) indeterminate CT findings, (4) renal vein or IVC not adequately visualized in other studies, (5) large tumor, or (6) preoperative embolization is desired. With the availability of digital subtraction technology, renal angiography can be done with smaller catheters, less contrast material, and thus often as an outpatient procedure.

IV digital subtraction angiography is valuable to determine the anatomy of the major renal vessels but has been proved to be of little value in the evaluation of the mass itself (Fig 2–12).[44, 45]

Venacavography

The use of abdominal venography in urologic disease dates back to the 1950s. Until recent years, it was the most reliable method available to identify and quantitate RCC tumor thrombi in the IVC. Although it is not necessary now, it had been recommended for use in every patient.[46] Even with the availability of ultrasonography and CT, we have relied on a venacavogram in patients who had large tumors, medial tumors, poor function of the kidney, or other symptoms that suggest IVC involvement. False-positive IVC results can be evident primarily from flow artifact from unopacified contrast material, distortion from the mass, or from involved lymph nodes. A normal venacavogram is presented in Figure 2–13, and it is easy to see how the flow artifact could potentially give the impression of a filling defect in the cava.

Magnetic Resonance Imaging

At this stage of development magnetic resonance imaging does not add significant additional information on the nature of the renal mass over CT. Logistic considerations, costs, long imaging time of the study, and restricted patient suitability (patients with pacemaker, intracranial aneurysm clip, life-support system, and most commonly, severe claustrophobia are excluded) make it

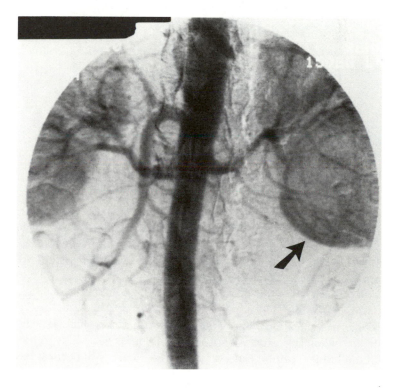

FIG 2–12.
IV digital subtraction angiography in a patient with a moderately sized left lower pole RCC (*arrow*). The renal arteries are well identified, but even though this is a hypervascular mass, it is poorly delineated on the IV digital subtraction angiography.

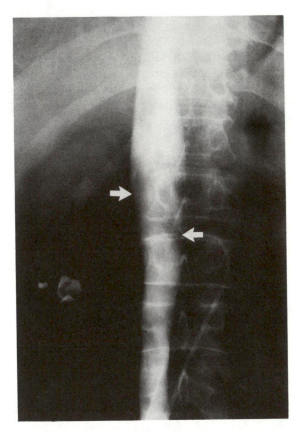

FIG 2–13.
Normal inferior venacavogram. *Arrows* indicate areas of flow of unopacified blood into the vena cava. In some situations this artifact can be confused with a filling defect in the vena cava.

unlikely that magnetic resonance imaging will be routinely used. A major application of magnetic resonance imaging is in the vascular aspects of RCC; the ability to study the patient in both transverse and coronal projections as well as with techniques highlighting various aspects of the vascular system are major advantages.

Radionuclide Scans

Radiopharmaceutical imaging of the kidney can occasionally be valuable in the evaluation of a mass lesion. An apparent solid mass, generally in the central portion of the kidney, can be caused by prominent areas of cortical tissue and have been termed *hypertrophied columns of Bertin, focal cortical hypertrophy, lobar dysmorphism,* and a *cortical island.*[47] Because this "mass" is composed of entirely normal renal tissue, a renal scan demonstrates normal function in the area of concern, differentiating it from a neoplasm that does not function

TABLE 2–5.
Renal Carcinomas in the Adult

TYPE	PERCENT
RCC	85
Transitional cell carcinoma of renal pelvis	10
Wilms' tumor	2
Other	3

normally. The radionuclides preferred now are technetium 99m-DMSA or glu-coheptonate.[47]

Imaging and Anatomic Pathology of Renal Cell Carcinoma

The purpose of this section is to describe various aspects of RCC, providing radiographic, gross, and histologic examples for correlation. Familiarity with often subtle radiographic findings and an understanding of the pathology that causes these findings make it easier to remember characteristic features and to be alert for the unusual case.

RCC is the most common renal malignancy representing 85% of all cases of cancer in the kidney (Table 2–5). Good communication between the urologist, radiologist, and pathologist requires that all appreciate what information is needed in the radiology and pathology reports. The following outline consists of variables that would be appropriately mentioned in the gross and microscopic pathologic description of the tumor.

I. Size.

II. Gross features.
  A. *Hemorrhage and necrosis.*
  B. *Cystic.*
  C. *Fibrous septa.*
  D. *Calcification.*

III. Stage.
  A. *Renal capsule and perinephric fat invasion.*
  B. *Intrarenal vascular invasion.*
  C. *Gross vascular invasion.*
  D. *Renal sinus invasion.*
  E. *Renal pelvis invasion.*
  F. *Lymph node invasion.*
  G. *Adjacent organ invasion.*

IV. Cell type.
  A. *Clear.*
  B. *Granular.*

    C. Sarcomatoid.
    D. Oncocytic.

 V. Growth pattern.

 VI. Nuclear grade.

 VII. Molecular abnormalities.

Some variables are important in defining prognosis. Others may be less significant, debatable, or of untested significance. As each variable is reviewed, data summarizing its value are presented. Additionally, examples of imaging aspects and gross and microscopic pathologic aspects of that particular variable are presented. Finally, the contribution of more recent technical advances, such as flow cytometry is discussed.

Some perspective on the pathology of RCC is appropriate. Confusion relative to the pathology of RCC dates back to the original descriptions. Grawitz in 1883 proposed that renal cancers arose from adrenal rests present in the renal cortex.[48] This was based on the then popular cell-rest theory of neoplasms and the gross similarities between renal cancers and a normal yellow-colored adrenal gland, thus the term *hypernephroma* or *Grawitz's tumor.* Sudek in 1893 proposed that renal adenocarcinoma arose from renal tubular cells; this dispute was not resolved until 1960 when Oberlin[48] confirmed by electron microscopy that the tumor arose from the proximal convoluted tubular cells in the kidney.

I. Size

The size of renal adenocarcinoma, generally recorded as the largest diameter, is a simple but noteworthy item in several aspects. From a tumor biology viewpoint, RCC is distinctive because of the large size frequently obtained in the absence of either symptoms or metastases. The average size of RCC is 6 to 7 cm, but tiny tumors are identified; it is common to have lesions greater than 10 cm still confined to the kidney (Fig 2–14).[48, 49] In other common epithelial carcinomas such as lung, breast, colon, or prostate cancer, a 7 cm tumor is an advanced local lesion and is likely to be associated with metastases. We mistakenly believed that RCC was often an aggressive cancer because 30% to 40% of patients have metastases. One, however, should compare the hazard of a similar RCC and prostate carcinoma (often believed to be an indolent carcinoma): a 7 cm renal carcinoma is usually confined to the kidney with a 10% to 20% chance of lymph node metastases, whereas a 7 cm prostate carcinoma would have lymph node metastases in 80% to 90% of cases and would likely be considered incurable.

The size of an RCC is a useful prognostic factor. For many years it was erroneously assumed that size was a reliable differential criterion between RCC and renal adenoma. Bell,[50] in a 1938 autopsy study, related size of the tumor to frequency of metastases, finding few metastases from lesions less than 3 cm (three of 65 or 4.6%). Unfortunately, interpretations of these data led to the concept that lesions less than 3 cm were benign, clearly not the case. As the size of the lesion increases, the progression of the local stage and the risk for metastases increase.[51] There is some evidence to suggest that large tumors may be seen less commonly than before, as demonstrated by the observation that approximately 10% of tumors now are greater than 10 to 12 cm versus 72% incidence in 1932 and a 30% to 40% incidence in 1950 to 1960.[49] This observation is logically attributed to earlier access to medical care and improved quality of imaging studies, specifically CT and ultrasonography. It has been suggested that this trend toward overall smaller tumors will translate into better survival.[52]

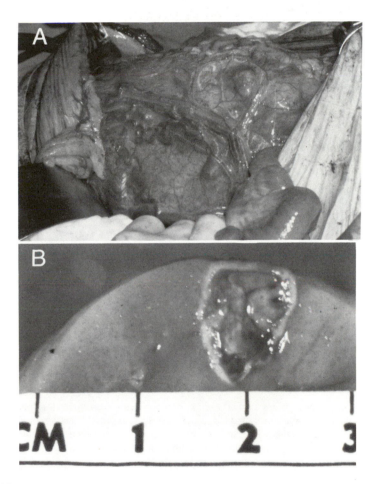

FIG 2–14.
A, approximately 25 cm right renal carcinoma occupying most of the entire abdomen in a 32-year-old woman. Initial complaint was shortness of breath resulting from a high output cardiac state, weight loss, and malaise. Dilated veins on the surface of the mass are apparent. **B,** tiny RCC slightly over 1 cm in diameter, which is microscopically indistinguishable from a typical RCC.

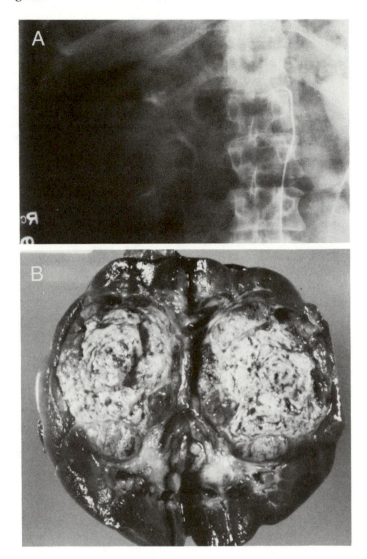

FIG 2–15.
A, IV urogram demonstrates distortion of the collecting system because of a mass located in the center of the normally functioning kidney. **B,** gross photograph of this tumor shows central location and distortion of the collecting system. This tumor is associated with a tumor thrombus that totally occludes the IVC and extends into the right atrium.

II. Gross Features

As noted earlier, the gross appearance of RCC contributed for many years to a fundamental error in understanding the origin of the tumor. The classic appearance is a yellow, round mass lesion, distorting the collecting system and adjacent parenchyma or protruding from the surface of the kidney (Figs 2–15 and 2–16). The yellow color is generally a reflection of lipid content, which is abundant in the common clear cell variant. Metastatic lesions also have a similar distinct color. Variations in the color to brown or tan correspond to predominance of granular or oncocytic cells and the amount of necrosis (Fig 2–17). Gray or gray-white areas have increased fibrosis.

Hemorrhage and Necrosis.—A common observation in RCC (present in approximately 90% of cases) is an extremely rich blood supply most readily demonstrated by arteriovenous "puddling" or shunting seen on angiography (Figs 2–18 to 2–20). The rich vascularity is associated with varying amounts of hemorrhage within the mass and often large areas of necrosis. This is a rather distinctive aspect of RCC, although poorly studied by tumor biologists. The degree of hemorrhage originating from a small tumor can be extensive and occasionally abrupt, leading to acute pain, mass, or a perirenal or retroperitoneal hematoma (Fig 2–2).[53] Areas of necrosis can occupy the majority of the tumor, necessitating care by the pathologist to microscopically examine areas that are

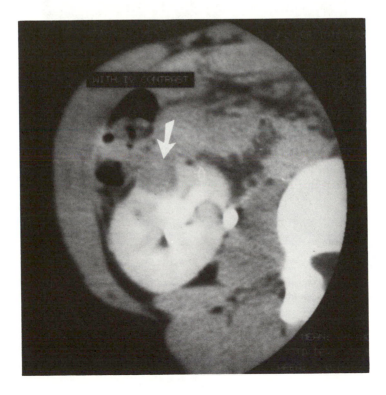

FIG 2–16.
CT scan demonstrates small mass protruding from surface of kidney. The mass was detected by palpation of the kidney during a gynecologic operation.

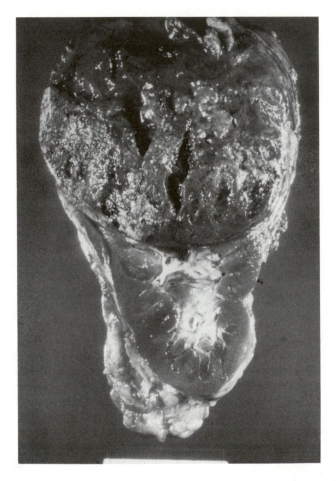

FIG 2–17.
Twelve-centimeter expansile, brown RCC of upper pole of kidney. Note appearance of fibrous capsule separating tumor from renal parenchyma.

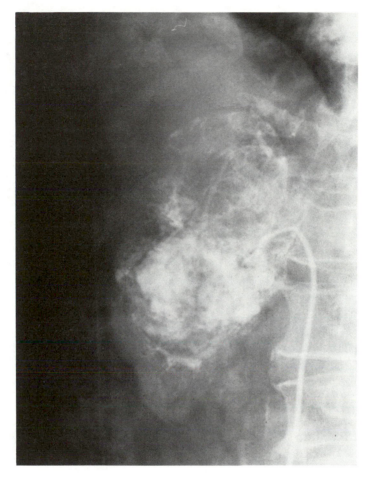

FIG 2–18.
Arteriogram demonstrates large amounts of "puddling" of contrast material as a result of intramural arteriovenous shunts. This is a characteristic appearance of RCC.

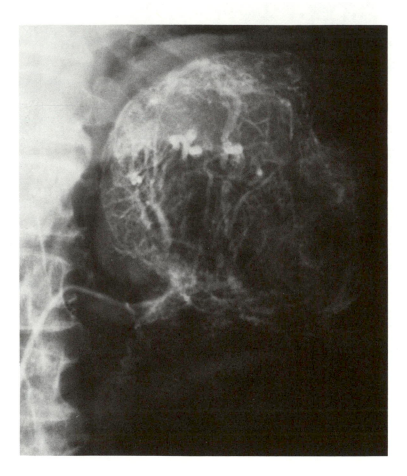

FIG 2–19.
Arteriogram of upper pole of left RCC demonstrates neovascularity with small aneurysm formation.

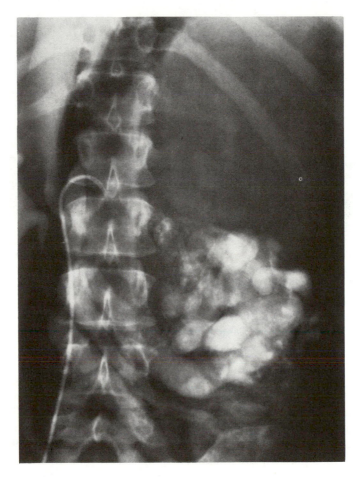

FIG 2–20.
Venous phase of renal arteriogram demonstrates marked arteriovenous shunts and collateral flow through large ovarian vein, which is distended and tortuous.

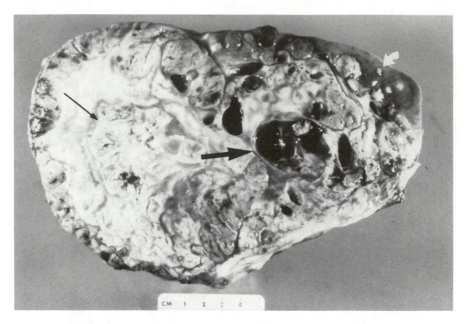

FIG 2–21.
Twenty-centimeter RCC with areas of necrosis and fibrosis (*thin black arrow*), extremely large intrarenal vein resulting from arteriovenous shunting within the tumor (*heavy black arrow*), and multiple satellite nodules (*white arrow*).

on the periphery of a necrotic area or that appear more viable (Fig 2–21). Tissue culture studies of RCC have often been hampered because adequate numbers of viable cells can be difficult to recover.

Cystic.—Large areas of necrosis in an RCC can lead to central liquefaction and to a cystic appearance. This is more commonly seen with large lesions and is appreciated preoperatively on urography, CT, or ultrasonography (Fig 2–22). The fluid in the cystic area is dark brown, pink, or "cheesy," providing a potential differential point from a simple cyst. Occasionally, an RCC can develop in the wall of a true simple cyst, and in this setting the tumor can be less obvious (Fig 2–23). The best example of this situation is seen in patients with von Hippel-Lindau disease in whom clear RCC cells can be seen microscopically lining the walls of an apparent simple cyst (Fig 2–24). Small carcinomas can be seen as a nodule in the cyst wall (Fig 2–25). Loculated cysts with a solid lesion in one area can present difficult diagnostic problems. The growth pattern of papillary adenocarcinoma can frequently be more grossly cystic, less vascular, and more necrotic, but may have a better prognosis.[54] In general, the amount of necrosis or vascularity of the tumor has not been linked to prognosis.

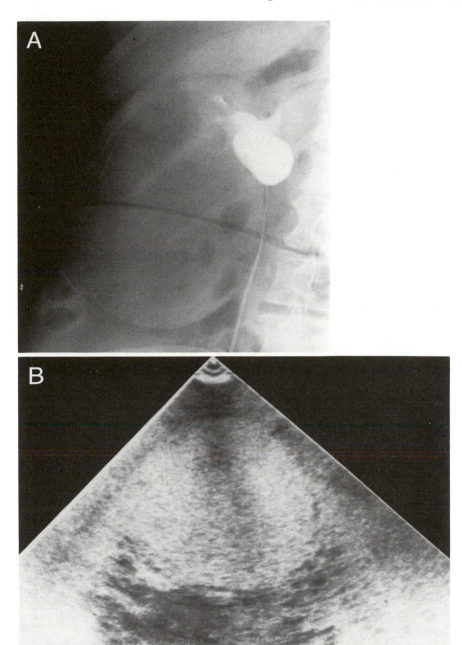

FIG 2–22.
A, IV pyelogram demonstrates large cystic mass in the lower pole of the right kidney. There is an apparent faint area of calcification in the rim seen in the lower aspect of the mass. **B,** longitudinal ultrasound examination demonstrates moderately echogenic mass. **C,** CT of this mass demonstrates heterogeneity in mass with areas of calcification.

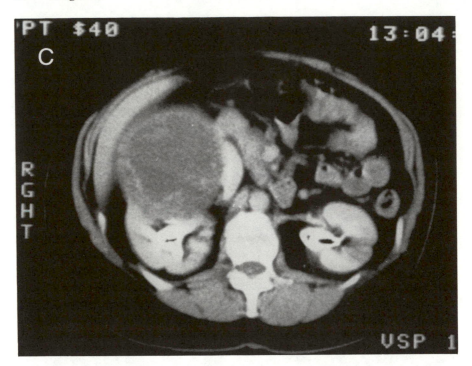

Fibrous Septa.—Fibrous septa are commonly seen in RCC, separating the mass into lobules. Occasionally a grossly apparent, dense desmoplastic response around the tumor can be seen, but the observation of this should raise suspicion of a sarcoma, malignant fibrous histiocytoma, or lymphoma. A fibrous "capsule" can be evident on gross examination, but multiple reports[55, 56] have confirmed the unreliability of this capsule as a barrier for true containment of the lesion (Fig 2–17). This is particularly relevant to the concept of enucleation, which has been used for some renal carcinomas. In this situation an incision in the cortex is made directly adjacent to the carcinoma, and then the lesion is "shelled out" away from the parenchyma. When this procedure has been examined carefully, up to 40% of cases have been found to have residual microscopic tumor, venous invasion, or capsular invasion that was not appreciated grossly.[55, 56]

Calcification.—The frequency of calcification in RCC depends on the method used to identify it. By gross examination focal calcification is seen in 15% to 20% of cases.[48, 49, 57] The pattern of calcification is a noteworthy observation relative to diagnostic studies but probably not a major variable relative to prognosis. In a classic article by Daniel et al,[58] nonperipheral or speckled calcification on an IVP was associated with malignancy in a large percentage of cases (80% to 90%) (Fig 2–22, A). A mass with rim calcification of the periphery has ap-

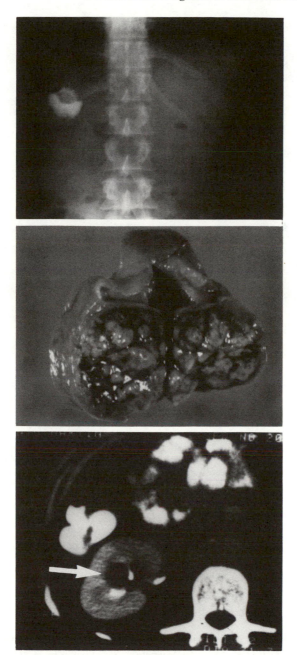

FIG 2–23.
Cystic lesion in central portion of right kidney identified on CT (*arrow*). Aspiration of this demonstrated pink fluid, and the cystogram showed an apparent filling defect on one wall. Gross specimens demonstrate solid neoplasm adjacent or arising from the wall of the cyst.

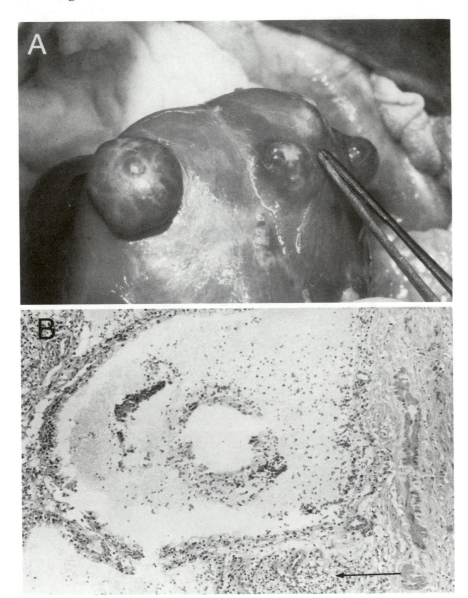

FIG 2–24.
von Hippel-Lindau disease. **A,** intraoperative photograph of multiple cortical cysts, each of which contains microscopic RCC. **B,** cyst lined by clear cell with underlying solid nest of RCC (*black arrow*). (Hematoxylin-eosin stain, magnification ×103.) **C,** cyst lined by flattened epithelium with cleared cytoplasm. (Hematoxylin-eosin stain, magnification ×206.)

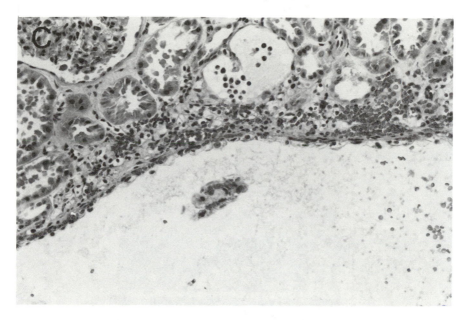

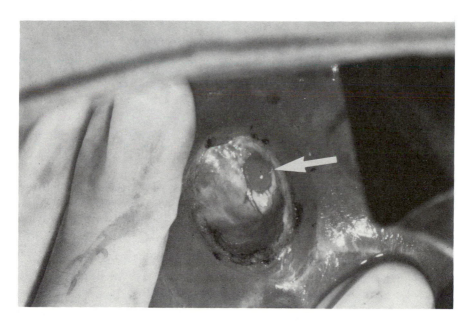

FIG 2–25.
Intraoperative photograph of patient with von Hippel-Lindau disease with small nodular tumor (*arrow*) arising from wall of what appears to be a typical cyst grossly.

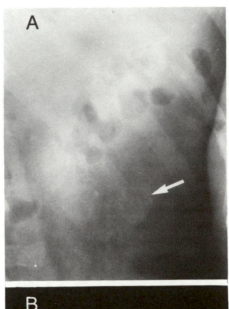

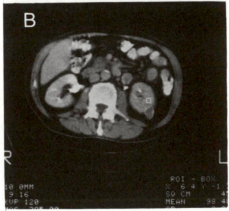

FIG 2–26.
A, preliminary abdominal film on a man who had an IV urogram for obstructive voiding symptoms. Small mass with rim calcification is noted on lateral aspect of the left kidney (*arrow*). **B,** CT of same patient demonstrates mass projecting off posterior lateral surface of the kidney with rim calcification evident. Histology identified RCC with perinephric fat invasion.

proximately a 20% chance of being malignant; additional diagnostic studies are needed to differentiate benign from malignant lesions. Calcification can frequently be identified by CT (Fig 2–26).

III. Stage
Although clinical studies provide needed information to identify metastases, the stage based on the local extent of the primary lesion is defined by the pathologist. Staging systems have been discussed in detail earlier in this chapter,

but it is important to emphasize again the reliance on the pathologist to provide the data that allow the appropriate stage to be assigned. Unlike many other carcinomas, clinical staging of the local lesion generally does not alter treatment decisions because surgical excision of RCC is the exclusive treatment.

Capsule and Perinephric Fat Invasion.—As early as 1932, Hand and Broder suggested that invasion of perinephric fat was associated with a shorter survival, 39 months versus 72 months.[48] Only approximately 30% of all RCCs are confined within the renal capsule. Invasion through the renal capsule can be either gross or microscopic, and yet the cancer is contained within Gerota's fascia; lesions in this group are classified as T_{3a} (American Joint Committee on Cancer, 1988) or stage II (Robson).[29, 31, 32] A major rationale for the routine use of a radical nephrectomy is the fact that this technique allows dissection outside of Gerota's fascia, thus all perinephric fat is removed (Fig 2–27). Gerota's fascia is an important barrier of tumor growth; penetration in this layer is uncommon and associated with large, locally advanced lesions that may invade colon, pancreas, or duodenum and are classified as T_4 (American Joint Committee on Cancer, 1988) or stage IV (Robson).[29–31]

Invasion of the renal capsule and then penetration into the perinephric fat can be seen with tumors of all sizes but clearly is more frequent with larger

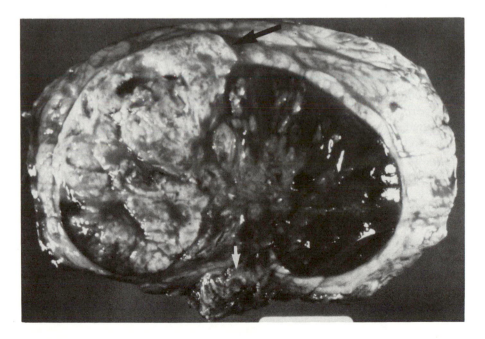

FIG 2–27.
RCC demonstrates invasion through renal capsule into perinephric fat (*black arrow*) but confined within Gerota's fascia (*black arrow*). Tumor thrombus evident in renal vein (*white arrow*).

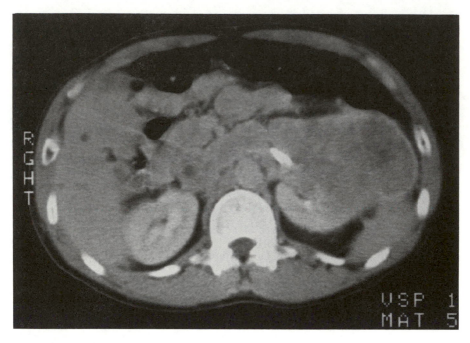

FIG 2–28.
CT scan demonstrates large loculated mass in the left kidney with involvement of the left renal vein extending into the IVC.

tumors. Careful gross and microscopic examination of the perinephric fat adjacent to the tumor is necessary, including examination of the renal sinus; Figure 2–26 is an example of a 2 cm carcinoma associated with microscopic invasion of the perinephric fat. Partial nephrectomy is commonly used for the treatment of selected cases of RCC, and excision of perinephric fat overlying the tumor and careful examination of this by the pathologist are important.

CT has been the best imaging study to evaluate the perinephric fat. Nevertheless, Johnson et al[59] found that CT correctly identified T_{3a} lesions in only 50% of cases, understandably because it is only a microscopic diagnosis in many cases. Angiography is particularly poor in the detection of perinephric fat invasion.[42]

Intrarenal Vascular Invasion.—Documentation of the extent of microscopic or gross intrarenal vascular invasion previously has not been considered an important variable. It is conceivable that a more critical appraisal of this variable would provide useful prognostic information, specifically in cases otherwise considered to be stage T_1 or T_2.[2]

Gross Vascular Invasion.—The propensity of RCC to invade large vascular channels is well established and is discussed at length in Chapter 5. Large venous thrombi can be identified in preoperative imaging studies (CT, ultrasonography, venacavogram, and magnetic resonance imaging) (Figs 2–28 to 2–30).[60, 61] False-positive results of studies on CT or venacavogram can be caused by flow artifacts. Smaller thrombi may not be evident to the radiologist or surgeon but must be identified by the pathologist (Fig 2–27). The venous phase of the angiogram can confirm an uninvolved renal vein (Fig 2–31). Gross vascular invasion has an adverse impact on survival to a similar degree afforded by perinephric fat invasion but not as bad as that afforded by lymph node invasion.[46, 49] The effect of the extent of venous involvement (i.e., renal vein alone versus several levels of IVC extension) is controversial with conflicting studies available (see Chapter 5). Precise documentation of the level of IVC extension requires the cooperation of the surgeon and the pathologist, and this information may be difficult to obtain in retrospective reviews.

Identification of renal venous or IVC invasion is important because the surgical approach may be modified. Renal vein invasion is identified by CT in 75% to 80% of involved cases. Dynamic scanning is helpful, but artifactual filling defects in the IVC can be seen from streaming or shunting of unopacified blood or distortion of the IVC from compression by the mass or enlarged lymph nodes (Fig 2–32). Although some authors believe CT or ultrasonography is adequate to define the upper extent of the IVC tumor thrombus, we have not been satisfied

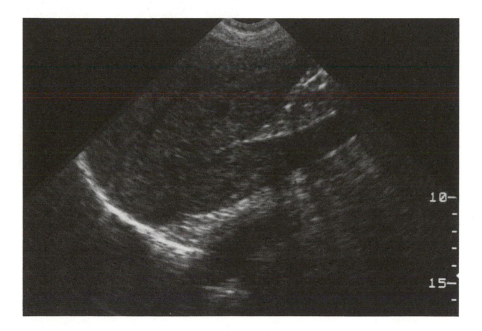

FIG 2–29.
Longitudinal thrombus in IVC identified by ultrasound examination.

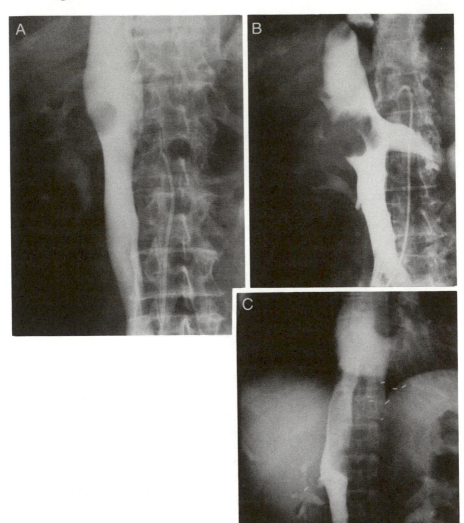

FIG 2–30.
A, inferior venacavogram demonstrates small (level 1) tumor thrombus evident by filling defect in contrast material. **B,** larger filling defect from tumor thrombus consistent with level 2 thrombus. There is no significant obstruction to the IVC. **C,** tumor thrombus and IVC from left-sided renal tumor. Thrombus extends at least up to the level of the diaphragm (level 3). Obstruction to the vena cava is not evident, and no collateral circulation is evident.

with this and generally use other techniques (Fig 2–33).[60] Angiography frequently demonstrates "arterialization" of the thrombus allowing detection and some degree of quantification (Fig 2–34). As noted earlier, magnetic resonance imaging offers a distinct advantage of allowing both transverse and coronal views to precisely define the extent of the thrombus.[61]

Controversy also exists relative to the importance of actual invasion of the IVC wall versus a free-floating or adherent thrombus. Conclusions are limited by little reliable data and the inability to control other variables that may be important. A concerted effort should be made to document the exact location of IVC invasion.

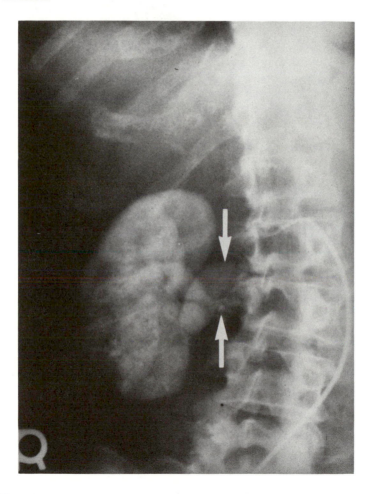

FIG 2–31.
Venous phase of renal arteriogram demonstrates early visualization of the renal vein (*arrows*) and confirms tumor thrombus is absent.

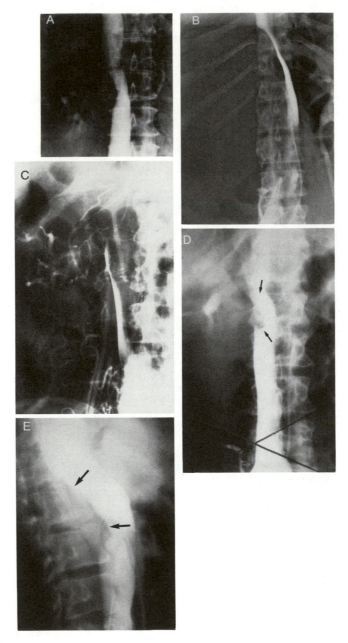

FIG 2–32.
Distortion of the IVC without intrinsic tumor thrombus. **A,** medial displacement of the cava resulting from compression from the right renal mass (*black arrows*). **B,** marked distortion and displacement as a result of large right renal mass. The cava was not invaded and was separated from the mass at operation. **C,** encasement of the vena cava with obstruction caused by large renal carcinoma. Resection of the cava was necessary. **D,** apparent filling defect in vena cava (*black arrows*) caused by distortion of the vena cava from hilar and retrocaval lymphadenopathy. **E,** lateral view of same case as **D** demonstrates anterior displacement of the vena cava from retrocaval lymph nodes that were identified on CT scan.

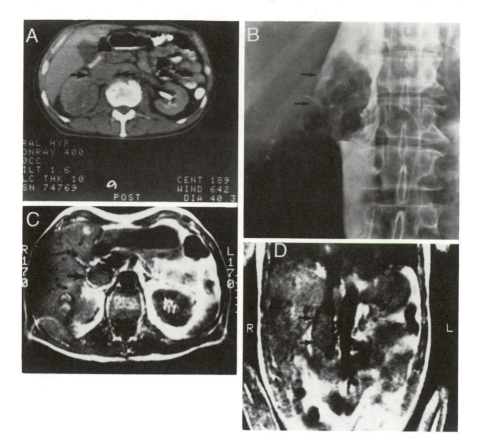

FIG 2–33.
Tumor thrombus in IVC demonstrated by various imaging methods in the same patient. **A,** CT scan demonstrates enlargement and obstruction of IVC (*black arrows*). **B,** inferior venacavogram demonstrates areas of involvement of vena cava with lobulated tumor thrombus (*black arrows*). **C,** transverse magnetic resonance imaging indicates presence of tumor thrombus in intrahepatic IVC (*black arrow*). **D,** coronal magnetic resonance imaging demonstrates tumor extension to the middle level of the intrahepatic IVC (*black arrows*), which shows uppermost extent.

Renal Sinus Invasion.—Contrary to evidence confirming the importance of renal sinus invasion with Wilms' tumor, no data are available to support the concept in RCC.[32, 49] Most studies, however, have been retrospective, and a systematic sampling of this area is often not accomplished. It is beneficial to include this information in the surgical pathology report.

Renal Pelvis Invasion.—Renal pelvis invasion has not been systematically evaluated but is not believed to be a significant prognostic factor.[49] An RCC invading the pelvis, however, can appear as a filling defect in the collecting system on contrast studies and thus can be confused clinically with a transitional cell carcinoma of the renal pelvis. The low frequency of gross renal pelvic invasion by RCC also contributes to the low frequency of malignant cells in the urine as detected by urine cytology studies.

Lymph Node Invasion.—Identification of retroperitoneal lymphadenopathy can be accomplished with CT, magnetic resonance imaging, or venacavogram (N + or stage III) (Fig 2–32, *D* and *E*).[31, 32] Lymph nodes greater than 2.0 cm or an increase in the number of lymph nodes are considered abnormal. Modest amounts of lymphadenopathy can be seen as a result of a benign inflammatory or immunologic response to the tumor. Before declaring a patient's condition inoperable or uncurable on the basis of lymphatic spread only, biopsy or fine needle aspiration is advisable. Magnetic resonance imaging may allow better delineation of relatively small nodes, but again these nodes may be either benign or malignant.

Approximately 25% of all patients with RCC will have involved nodes. If only patients without other metastatic sites are considered, the incidence decreases to 10% to 15%.[62]

Involvement of regional lymph nodes by RCC is universally accepted as indicative of a poor prognosis.[62] Debate, however, is evident in several areas

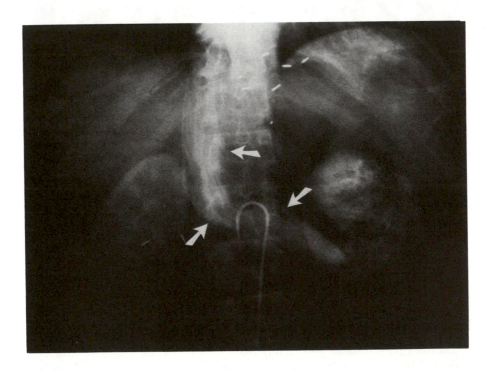

FIG 2–34.
"Arterialization" of tumor thrombus in left renal vein and IVC extending up to the diaphragm (*white arrows*).

relative to dissection of the nodes. Robson advocated extensive node dissection around the ipsilateral great vessel (IVC or aorta) as a means of improving survival.[29] Because his results with radical nephrectomy were superior to historical data, the lymphadenectomy was accepted by many as the reason responsible for the better results. Two observations, however, make this conclusion uncertain. First, regional lymphatic drainage from the kidney can be quite variable, involving iliac nodes or interaortic caval nodes as initial draining sites in addition to pericaval or precaval (right-sided tumor) and periaortic or preaortic nodes (left-sided tumor).[63] To remove all potentially involved nodes requires a substantial dissection. Second, 5-year survival of patients with nodal metastases is poor, generally estimated to be 10% to 20%.[62] In the Cleveland Clinic experience, long-term disease-free survival was unusual in patients with positive nodes and was restricted to patients with isolated or microscopic disease located in renal hilar nodes.[63–65] Thus we have not advocated such an extensive dissection as have others.[63, 65]

Thus the pathologist's examination of regional lymph nodes is dependent on the extent of dissection performed. In any event the pathologist must carefully examine the renal hilar region to look for lymph nodes.

Adjacent Organs.—The most common adjacent organ involved with RCC is the ipsilateral adrenal gland. Historically metastases or direct extension were noted in up to 10% of surgical cases.[66] This observation is the rationale for the accepted surgical practice of resection of the ipsilateral adrenal gland as an integral part of a radical nephrectomy. More recently, Robey and Schellhammer[66] have emphasized that adrenal involvement may be less frequent (2%) and is usually seen with large or upper pole carcinomas, thus the adrenal gland need not be removed in all cases. Contralateral only or bilateral adrenal involvement is occasionally seen but is usually evident preoperatively on imaging studies.

Identification of invasion of other organs is extremely difficult with CT. Tissue planes between the mass and the liver, colon, or duodenum can be completely obliterated without direct extension of the carcinoma into these organs (Fig 2–35). Direct invasion of the liver is extremely rare. Vascular mass lesions in the liver may not necessarily be a metastasis or a direct extension because liver hemangiomas have a similar appearance and are quite common.

Penetration through Gerota's fascia is a late occurrence in RCC; the tumor can invade directly into colonic mesentery, colon, duodenum, tail of pancreas, spleen, or diaphragm and is then classified as T_4 (American Joint Committee on Cancer) or stage IV (Robson).[31, 32] Although prognosis is admittedly poor in these circumstances, resection is needed in selected cases.

IV. Cell Type

A large amount of literature is available describing the morphology and significance of different cell types in RCC. Neither the classic clear cell type or granular cell type influences prognosis significantly when other variables are

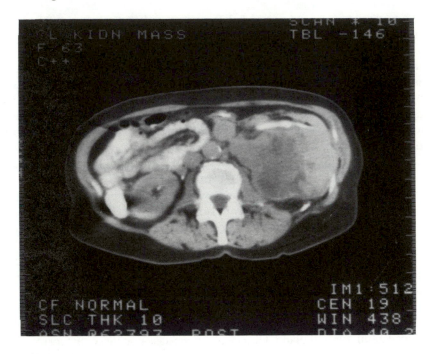

FIG 2–35.
CT scan of left RCC illustrates complete loss of anterior fat planes between the surface of the kidney and the overlying colon and small bowel. None of the bowel was involved with this lesion, and the tumor was resected entirely.

controlled.[48, 67, 68] The more recently described sarcomatoid morphology worsens prognosis. Most tumors are mixtures of more than one cell type, predominantly clear and granular cells.

Clear Cell.—The predominance of clear carinoma cells is seen in 50% to 60% of tumors; it has been appreciated since the earliest description of RCC. The clear cells are rich in lipid and/or glycogen demonstrable by periodic acid-Schiff stain, giving the classic yellow color grossly and the clear cytoplasm microscopically (Fig 2–36). The cell of origin is the proximal convoluted tubule cell. Electron microscopy shows a low density of organelles. The clear cell morphology in a biopsy specimen of a metastasis occasionally allows identification of the kidney as the primary site of the tumor. No specific imaging characteristic separates a clear cell from a granular cell lesion.

Granular Cell.—Tumors composed predominantly of granular cells are less common, identified in 15% to 25% of cases (Fig 2–37). The granular appearance of the cytoplasm is caused by a high density of organelles, primarily mitochondria, which can be identified by electron microscopy. Although the granular cell has less lipid than the clear cell, it also arises from the proximal convoluted tubule and produces numerous microvilli on the cell surface.

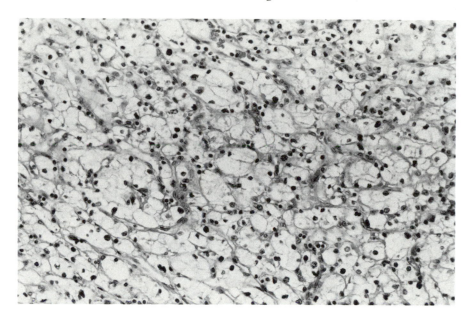

FIG 2–36.
Clear cell type of RCC. The tumor cells contain clear cytoplasm and grades I to II nuclei.
(Hematoxylin-eosin stain, magnification ×206.)

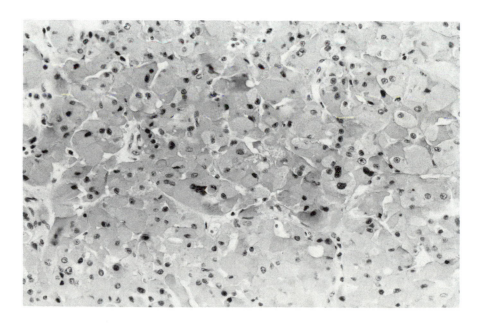

FIG 2–37.
Granular cell type of RCC, nuclear grade II. (Hematoxylin-eosin stain, magnification ×206.)

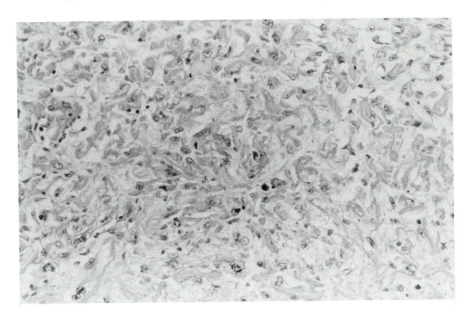

FIG 2–38.
Sarcomatoid RCC. Elongated tumor cells show no definite characteristics of RCC. (Hematoxylin-eosin stain, magnification ×206.)

Sarcomatoid.—The sarcomatoid morphology is uncommon as a predominant cell type (1% of cases) but is nonetheless important to appreciate.[69] Noted in the 1960s by Farrow, this cell type is associated with a distinct adverse effect on prognosis, with the local lesion often being more extensive and the risk of metastases higher than with a typical RCC.[69] There are sheets of spindle cells, possibly in a whorled pattern, which can abut or intermingle with more typical carcinomatous areas (Fig 2–38). Numerous mitoses and multiple giant cells are common. Ultrastructural studies[70] may be helpful in confirming the underlying diagnosis of RCC. On imaging studies[71] the tumors tend to be slightly less vascular on angiography but are quite locally extensive on CT.

Oncocytic.—The characteristics of the classic oncocytoma as a distinct entity are discussed later. Some tumors, however, contain areas composed of varying amounts of cells that have been termed *oncocytic*.[72] These cells are typified by a large uniform granular cytoplasm that is extremely rich in mitochondria, even to a denser level than the granular cell type.

V. Growth Pattern

A considerable degree of inconsistency appears when growth patterns are described. Descriptive terms such as solid and/or granular, papillary, papillary cystic, tubular, spindled acinar, alveolar, and sarcomatoid have been used.[48, 49, 68]

It is likely that the architectural growth pattern provides little prognostic significance with the exception of two categories. A spindled or sarcomatoid pattern composed of cells arranged in organized bundles or sheets is associated with the cell type described earlier as sarcomatoid and is consistently linked to a poor prognosis. Conversely, a papillary pattern has been classically associated with a more favorable prognosis, although contradictory data are available (Fig 2–39).[49, 54] The papillary growth pattern has been associated commonly with a low local stage, high frequency of calcification, less enhancement on CT, and relative hypovascularity on angiography (Fig 2–40).[54, 73]

VI. Grade

Nuclear grading systems have not been widely accepted, although multiple reports[51, 69, 72] have demonstrated some influence on prognosis in cases at either end of the spectrum. Petersen[49] believes that grading systems based on nuclear features do not adequately stratify most cases of RCC. No protocols available have been proved reproducible, thus it is difficult to recommend a grading system that should be utilized.[48, 49, 51, 68, 69, 74] The recognition of cases at each end of the spectrum, however, is probably valuable. The grading criteria used at the Cleveland Clinic are listed in Table 2–6.

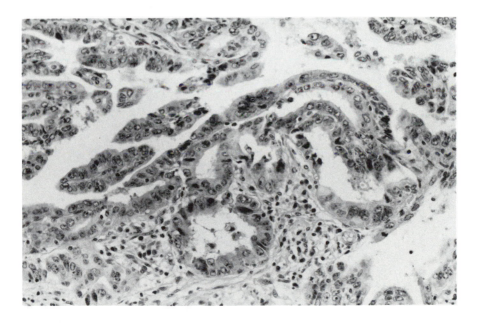

FIG 2–39.
Papillary RCC. Neoplastic glands and papillary formation is at left of center. Tumor contains enlarged irregular cells with nucleolated nuclei. (Hematoxylin-eosin stain, magnification ×206.)

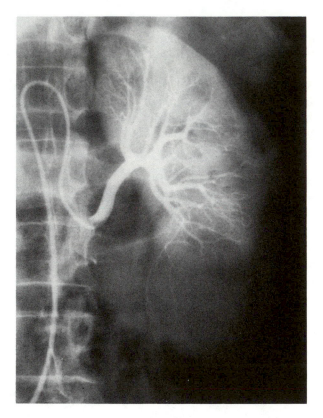

FIG 2–40.
Arteriogram of papillary RCC demonstrates typical hypovascularity of this growth pattern. A few small abnormal vessels can be seen coursing to the carcinoma.

TABLE 2–6.
Nuclear Grade*

GRADE	SIZE
1	10 μm nuclei, inconspicuous nucleoli
2	15 μm nuclei, nucleoli
3	20 μm irregular nuclei, prominent nucleoli
4	Similar to grade 3 with multilobed nuclei and hyperchromatism, includes sarcomatoid tumors

*Adapted from Fuhrman SA, Lasky LC, Limas C: *Am J Surg Pathol* 1982; 6:655–663.

VII. Molecular Abnormalities

Several studies[75, 76] have identified specific chromosome alterations on the short arm of chromosome 3 in nonfamilial RCC. As technical advances allow easier and more precise dissection of the cellular deoxyribonucleic acid (DNA) makeup, more information such as this will be available and may be of considerable importance.

The development of monoclonal antibodies to RCC is another technologic advance that may be proved clinically useful.[77, 78] It is possible that some tumor-associated antigens may exist with specificity that would allow monoclonal antibodies directed against tumor-associated antigens to be valuable in diagnosis or detection of metastases. The use of monoclonal antibodies bound to radioisotopes suitable for nuclear medicine imaging or therapy is being explored.[79]

Similar to many other carcinomas, progress in understanding the genetic abnormalities of cancer cells has stimulated the use of improved technology to study individual cases. Abnormalities in nuclear DNA content, either by karyotyping or flow cytometry have been studied by several authors.[76, 80, 81] Preliminary studies suggest that RCC will follow a pattern like other carcinomas: The more severe the genetic distortion in the cell (i.e., aneuploid cell lines and abnormal marker chromosomes), the worse the prognosis. How widely these findings can be reproduced and how well these observations compare with other prognostic measurements remain to be studied.

In summary, vital information relative to prognosis is provided by the pathologist. Stage is the most important variable, but certain growth patterns and histologic features are also noteworthy. If an effective adjuvant systemic therapy becomes available, a more exhaustive multivariate analysis on a large cohort of patients will be needed to better quantify the later risk of metastases. Unfortunately, the lack of comparable and complete reporting methods makes an analysis such as this currently impossible.

Well-differentiated tumors with uniform small size and round shape of nuclei with inconspicuous nucleoli, which demonstrate little mitotic activity should be noted.[72] Commonly these findings would be seen in a small tumor that does not invade the capsule and thus would be anticipated to be less dangerous. On the other extreme, tumors that are pleomorphic and barely recognizable as RCC are generally aggressive. Most cases (80% to 90%) do not fit into either of these categories; thus the value of nuclear grading is debatable.

Imaging and Anatomic Pathology in the Differential Diagnosis of RCC

The differential diagnosis of RCC is provided in the following outline.

  I. Benign.
     A. *Adenoma.*
     B. *Oncocytoma.*
     C. *Angiomyolipoma.*
     D. *Xanthogranulomatous pyelonephritis, malakoplakia, renal abscess.*

E. *Cystic disease.*
1. Simple cyst with hemorrhage.
2. Cysts in von Hippel-Lindau disease.
3. Acquired renal cystic disease.
4. Polycystic kidney disease.
5. Multilocular cyst.
F. *Renal medullary interstitial tumor.*
G. *Hemangioma and lymphangioma.*
H. *Juxtaglomerular cell tumor.*
I. *Capsular and perirenal lesions.*

II. Malignant.
A. *Lymphoproliferative malignancies.*
B. *Epithelial tumors of renal pelvis.*
C. *Adult Wilms' tumor.*
D. *Metastatic carcinoma to kidney.*
E. *Adrenocortical carcinoma.*
F. *Sarcomas.*

Commonly, a urologist, with clues from the radiologic evaluation, can alert the pathologist to the potential for the difficulty in diagnosis based on some peculiar aspects in the clinical situation. These clues are discussed along with the lesions.

I. Benign Lesions

Adenoma.—Small, nodular cortical lesions in the kidney have been recognized for almost 100 years and were originally thought to be adrenal rests. Later studies[82] demonstrated that these lesions were common, occurring in 7% to 23% of autopsy studies and 17% in a surgical series of RCC by Makamel et al.[82] The often quoted (or misquoted) work by Bell has been mentioned previously.[50] The rather arbitrary size differential of 3 cm diameter was chosen because few (but not zero) lesions this size or smaller metastasized. Data accumulated since then clearly show that size is not an appropriate measurement to distinguish benign from malignant tumors, although smaller lesions are generally less aggressive than larger lesions.[48, 49, 51]

One would assume that the distinction between adenoma and carcinoma would be resolved on histologic, histochemical, and or ultrastructural grounds; this has not been the case. Bennington and Beckwith[48] and Petersen[49] believe that no definite distinctions are possible, thus the term *renal adenocarcinoma of low metastatic potential* should be used for these small lesions. Mostofi and Davis[83] have described specific characteristics of papillary adenomas believed to be truly benign (Fig 2–41). On a practical basis small solid lesions in the parenchyma of the kidney should be treated as potentially malignant and excised totally, either by total or partial nephrectomy, and not just sampled for biopsy because of the above concerns and sampling considerations (see Chapter 6).

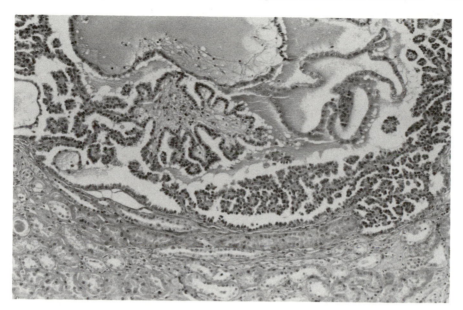

FIG 2–41.
Papillary adenoma. Unencapsulated neoplastic papillary formation lined by flattened, and cuboidal cells without anaplasia. (Hematoxylin-eosin stain, magnification × 103.)

Oncocytoma.—The renal lesion termed *oncocytoma* has been recognized widely after Klein and Valensi described 13 cases in 1976.[84] Their retrospective review of a large number of cases of RCC from one institution identified a subset of patients with tumors that have the following typical features: (1) well-demarcated borders; (2) mahogany brown color; (3) variable size but occasionally quite large; (4) stellate central scar, often seen on CT or magnetic resonance imaging; (5) monotonous pattern of large granular eosinophilic cells arranged in tubules with small regular nuclei, sharp borders, and virtually no mitoses; (6) characteristic pattern on electron microscopy with many mitochondria and a well-developed endoplasmic reticulum; and (7) usually associated with no symptoms (Fig 2–42).[84, 85] This classic lesion is believed to be benign and a form of adenoma. A dilemma, however, is evident because some RCCs have areas of what has been termed *oncocytic appearance,* different grades of oncocytomas have been described; some tumors that are apparently oncocytomas have small foci of frank carcinoma, some oncocytomas have karyotypic abnormalities, some tumors designated as oncocytomas have metastasized, and oncocytomas can coexist with RCC in the same or contralateral kidney.[84–86] Although several characteristics on imaging studies can suggest the diagnosis of oncocytoma, it is unlikely that they are specific enough to obviate surgical excision of the mass. The central scar seen on magnetic resonance imaging or CT can also be seen in RCC (Fig 2–43). Angiographically, oncocytomas have classically had a "spoke-wheel" pattern with a central avascular area from the central scar. Necrosis in

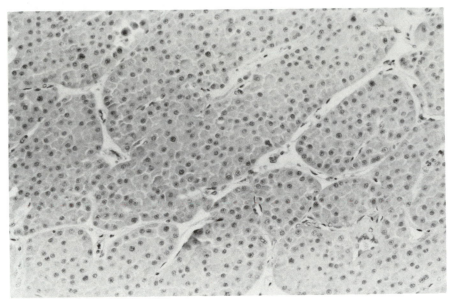

FIG 2–42.
Oncocytoma. Solid nest of uniform cells with small round nuclei and granular cytoplasm. (Hematoxylin-eosin stain, magnification ×206.)

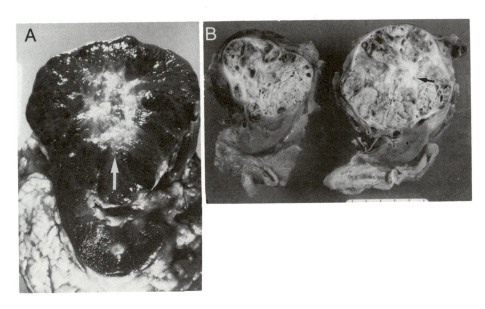

FIG 2–43.
Differentiation of oncocytoma versus RCC. **A,** brown homogeneous oncocytoma with typical central scar (*white arrow*). **B,** moderately homogeneous tumor demonstrates central scar (*black arrow*). This turned out to be an RCC, and appearance on CT scan was essentially identical to oncocytoma in **A.**

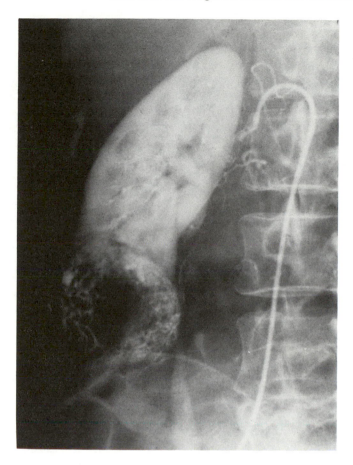

FIG 2–44.
Renal arteriogram of mass in lower pole of right kidney demonstrates neovascularity in large area of central avascularity consistent with a central scar. This proved to be an RCC.

RCC, however, can also have a similar appearance (Fig 2–44). On the basis of all of the above variables oncocytoma should be a diagnosis established only after the mass has been excised completely. Radiographic diagnoses may be erroneous, and diagnosis made on the basis of a biopsy or fine needle aspiration only may not be representative of all areas of the tumor. It is important that all criteria of diagnosis be satisfied, particularly in regard to nuclear size and shape. The nuclei should resemble those of adjacent nonneoplastic proximal convoluted tubule cells.

Angiomyolipoma.—An angiomyolipoma is a benign renal tumor with varying amounts of three histologic components: abnormal blood vessels, poorly organized smooth muscle cells that develop from vessel walls or grow in sheets,

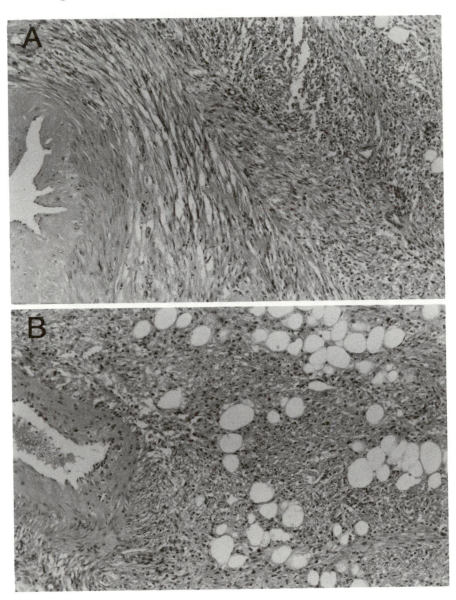

FIG 2–45.
Angiomyolipoma. **A,** thick wall blood vessel (*left*), fascicles of smooth muscle (*center*), and occasional fat cells (*right*). (Hematoxylin-eosin stain, magnification ×103.) **B,** blood vessel (*left*) with fascicles of smooth muscle developing from the wall and clusters of fat cells. (Hematoxylin-eosin stain, magnification ×103.)

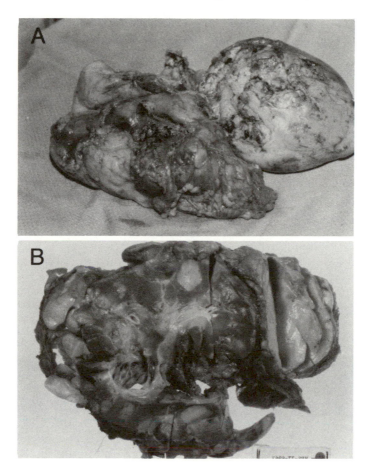

FIG 2–46.
A, gross specimen of large angiomyolipoma demonstrates nodules in the kidney and a large mass projecting off the kidney. **B,** angiomyolipoma with more prominent involvement in the cortex and multiple nodules.

and mature adipose tissue (Fig 2–45).[48, 49] The lesion was originally described as part of the tuberous sclerosis complex also including mental retardation, epilepsy, and adenoma sebaceum. An estimated 50% to 80% of patients with tuberous sclerosis have renal angiomyolipoma, often bilateral, multiple, and sometimes with renal cysts (Fig 2–46).[87] The lesions are benign hamartomas. Unfortunately, RCC may be seen in this patient population, and clinical differentiation between the two lesions can be problematic. Rarely patients have both angiomyolipoma and RCC.

Angiomyolipoma is actually seen more commonly as an isolated entity in the kidney in the absence of tuberous sclerosis, especially in women.[87, 88] The lesion can vary in size but commonly can be symptomatic and large, destroying the kidney and expanding into the perinephric fat and even into lymph nodes and the renal vein. Hemorrhage in the lesion can be sudden and life-threatening, occasionally necessitating emergent intervention (Fig 2–47).

An angiomyolipoma should be suspected when areas of fat in the mass are seen on the abdominal CT scan, when the angiogram demonstrates a typical "onion-peel" appearance on the venous phase, when bilateral lesions are seen, and in patients with tuberous sclerosis (Fig 2–48). Unfortunately, areas of necrosis in RCC can appear as low density on a CT scan, RCC can be bilateral, and it can also be seen in patients with tuberous sclerosis. Observation only is acceptable treatment for selected angiomyolipomas based on classic radiographic findings; if there is any doubt, excision is wise either with a partial or total nephrectomy.[88] Because these lesions are invariably benign, in many instances it is wise to attempt to conserve renal parenchyma. The natural history of angiomyolipoma is also variable with expansile growth seen in some and minimal progression in others.

If clinical circumstances suggest an angiomyolipoma, the pathologist should be forewarned. Biopsy of the lesion can be complicated by severe hemorrhage

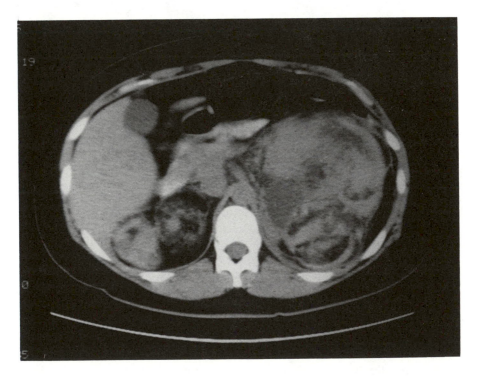

FIG 2–47.
Bilateral angiomyolipoma with hemorrhage on the left side. Areas of decreased attenuation on the left are not typical of fat and are more consistent with necrosis or hemorrhage.

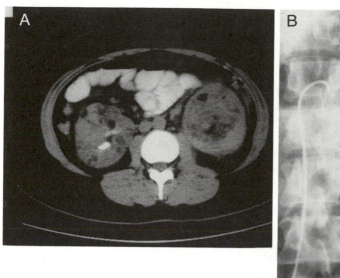
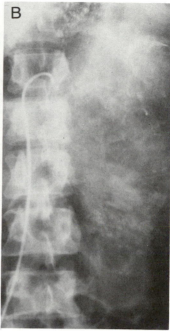

FIG 2–48.
A, CT demonstrates bilateral angiomyolipoma with more typical areas of low attenuation from fat in neoplasm. **B,** late phase of arteriogram demonstrates marked hypervascularity of angiomyolipoma. Arteriographic findings can suggest a differentiation between RCC and angiomyolipoma but are not conclusive.

because of the abnormal vasculature and difficult pathologic identification of all three histologic elements. Some lesions will have little or no fat and histologically are angiomyomas.

Xanthogranulomatous Pyelonephritis, Malacoplakia, and Renal Abscess.— Xanthogranulomatous pyelonephritis, malacoplakia, and renal abscess are three benign inflammatory conditions that can easily appear as mass lesions in the kidney and be confused with RCC on clinical, gross, and microscopic examinations.[48]

Xanthogranulomatous pyelonephritis, first described in 1916 by Schlagenhaufer, is characterized histologically by the presence of large numbers of foamy macrophages (histiocytes), resulting in a yellow color resembling clear cell RCC.[49] Although inflammatory in origin, it can appear clinically as a symptomatic, large nodular lesion and involve the perinephric tissue and even adjacent bowel (Fig 2–49). Aspects differentiating this from RCC include an extremely common association with hydronephrosis, fever, urinary tract infection (UTI) with gram-negative sepsis, and renal calculi, often staghorn.[89] Grossly, the kidney shows a ragged hydronephrosis with extensive destruction of the collecting system. The inner zone of the collecting system is necrotic. The next peripheral zone is yellow because of lipid in histiocytes, and the outer zone is pale gray due to fibrosis and inflammation. This classic appearance is nontransmural and is zonal in character. Microscopically, areas of gross pus can be seen in the collecting system with an inflammatory response in adjacent parenchyma, composed of many histiocytes. Generally, nephrectomy is needed even if the diagnosis is appreciated preoperatively. Rarely, drainage with removal of the urinary obstruction and stones, followed by administration of antibiotics, is sufficient if need be and can be done if preservation of renal parenchyma is needed. Most often, however, there is massive loss of renal parenchyma.

Malacoplakia is a rare inflammatory condition that can occur in many organs

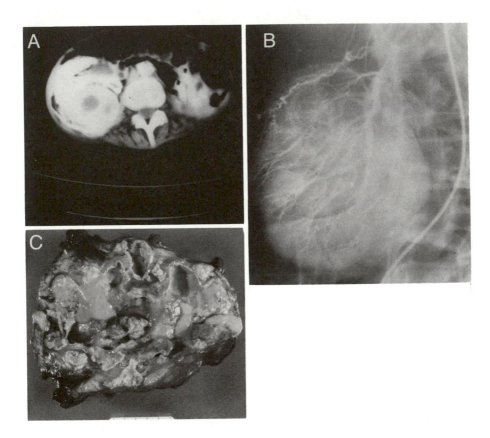

FIG 2–49.
Xanthogranulomatous pyelonephritis. **A,** CT scan indicates large complex mass in posterior aspect of the right kidney. **B,** arteriogram demonstrates hypervascularity in abnormal vessels of previous mass. **C,** gross photograph of excised kidney illustrates areas of gross pus formation and calculi.

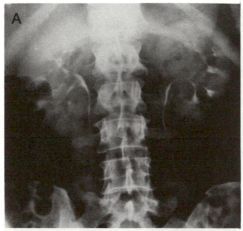
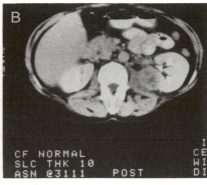
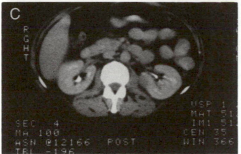

FIG 2–50.
A, IV urogram of 45-year-old woman with acute left flank pain and one episode of fever. No source of infection was apparent. **B,** CT scan in same patient demonstrates complex mass in posteromedial aspect of the left kidney with thickening of the psoas muscle. This degree of abnormality in the psoas muscle adjacent to a relatively small tumor would be unlikely and raised the suspicion of an inflammatory process. **C,** CT scan (24 days after antibiotic therapy is administered) demonstrates almost complete resolution of the mass.

in addition to the kidney.[90] Pathologically, it is composed of large histiocytes and areas of necrosis, grossly appears as a plaque in the collecting system, but occasionally has a yellow or tan nodular lesion in the parenchyma.[48, 49] The characteristic feature is cytoplasmic inclusions within histiocytes termed *Michaelis-Gutmann bodies,* which are laminated calcific bodies. These are believed to arise through phagocytosis of bacteria by histiocytes. Clinically, the lesion is usually seen in female patients who have some compromise in their immune system, which can be caused by diabetes, organ transplantation, alcoholism, or chronic urinary tract infection.

An uncomplicated renal abscess can appear as a mass lesion on imaging studies, including angiography, and may mimic RCC (Fig 2–50). An acute onset of symptoms with fever might suggest the diagnosis. Antibiotic therapy with or without aspiration of the lesion diminishes or eliminates the mass allowing confirmation of the diagnosis of the benign process.

Cystic Disease.—Multiple types of cysts can represent diagnostic dilemmas and must be distinguished from RCC.

Simple Cyst With Hemorrhage.—Occasionally a simple cyst may appear to be a malignancy because of hemorrhage into the cyst. Preoperative differentiation is not feasible, and these lesions must be explored. CT and ultrasonography will show a cystic mass with a more dense fluid internally. Angiography will not demonstrate tumor vessels, but this will not eliminate the possibility of a carcinoma. Magnetic resonance imaging and aspiration of the mass both show blood, either relatively fresh or old and organized. Excision of the mass is probably the safest approach if this is technically feasible (Fig 2–51). Unroofing of the cyst is not the ideal treatment, since the small tumor at the base may not be visible or difficult to identify on a frozen section.

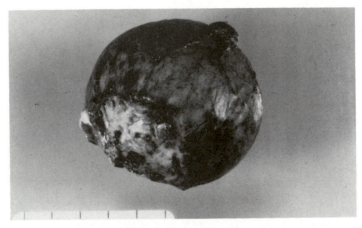

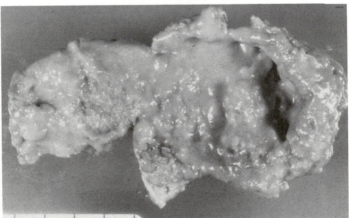

FIG 2–51.
Renal cyst with hemorrhage. Photograph of gross specimen of excised renal cyst filled with old, organizing, hematoma. Multiple sections in the cyst wall were negative for carcinoma.

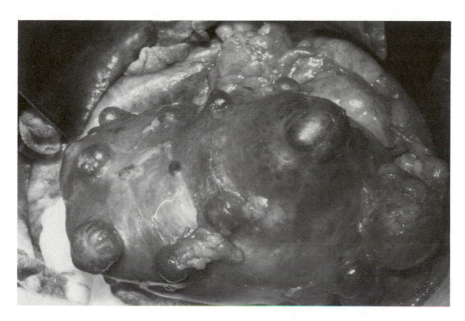

FIG 2–52.
von Hippel-Lindau disease. Bilateral solid and cystic renal masses. There were multiple cysts present in both kidneys, many of which were not appreciated on CT scan.

Cysts in von Hippel-Lindau Disease.—As noted earlier, von Hippel-Lindau disease is the constellation of abnormalities including RCC (often bilateral multiple abnormalities occurring at an early age), multiple renal, epididymal, pancreatic cysts, retinal hemangiomas, cerebellar and spinal cord hemangioblastomas, and pheochromocytomas. The cysts in the kidney in this entity must be suspect for RCC, especially in someone with known RCC (see Figs 2–24 and 2–25). Attempts at conservative surgery have been made, but once a pattern of multifocal disease develops, nephrectomies probably will be needed at some time (see Chapter 4).[91] We believe that the renal cysts lined by clear epithelium are incipient RCC.

CT and angiography vastly underestimate the number of cysts; carcinomas can only be detected by ultrasonography, CT, or magnetic resonance imaging when they become large enough to be visualized (Fig 2–52).

Acquired Renal Cystic Disease.—Acquired renal cystic disease is a newly recognized entity seen with increasing frequency. Described by Dunnell in 1977, acquired renal cystic disease is seen in patients receiving long-term dialysis therapy with the frequency increasing with time on dialysis and with a prevalence of 40% to 80%.[92, 93] The development of RCC in up to 25% of patients in this setting, often starting as papillary projections from the epithelial lining of the cyst is noteworthy.[49, 93] Periodic ultrasonic or CT scan examination of the kidneys is needed in patients receiving chronic dialysis; further evaluation is warranted if there is suspected transformation of a cyst into a complex, solid, or enlarging lesion (Fig 2–53).

Adult Polycystic Kidney Disease.—Adult polycystic kidney disease is a predominantly inherited disease characterized by large renal and hepatic cysts. Progression to renal failure is common, but development of azotemia is variable. Hemorrhage into these cysts is common, and differentiation from a solid mass can be problematic. CT, magnetic resonance imaging, and angiography can provide valuable information (Fig 2–54).

Multilocular Cyst (Multilocular Cystic Nephroma).—Multilocular cyst is a rare cystic disorder of the kidney and has a debated origin. As a loculated lesion evident on CT, magnetic resonance imaging, or ultrasonography, differentiation from an RCC with cystic areas or RCC in the wall of the cyst can be extremely difficult clinically (Fig 2–55). The lesion occurs in infants and young boys and in older adults, generally women.

If a multilocular cyst is suspected, surgical removal by a partial nephrectomy if feasible, is recommended. Careful sampling by the pathologist of multiple areas of each of the cysts is appropriate and should identify a benign epithelium

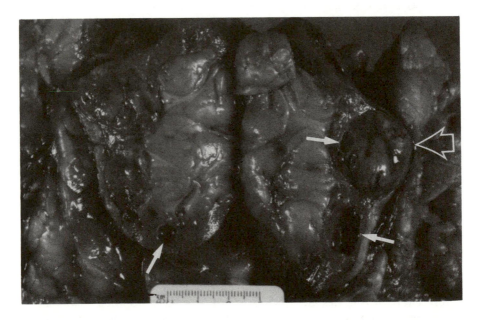

FIG 2–53.
Acquired renal cystic disease. *Open arrow* indicates solid RCC in the cortex. *Closed white arrows* indicate multiple renal cysts, including one directly adjacent to the solid mass. Of note is severe loss of renal parenchyma associated with chronic renal failure from glomerulonephritis.

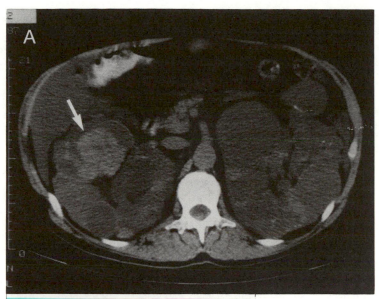

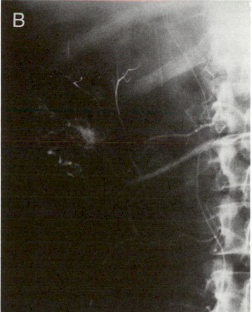

FIG 2–54.
Polycystic kidney disease with RCC. **A,** CT shows area of increased enhancement in anterior portion of right kidney (*white arrow*). Remainder of kidneys demonstrate typical findings of polycystic disease. **B,** right renal arteriogram in this patient demonstrates an area of hypervascularity in the area of the malignancy and other areas typical of splaying of the vessels from polycystic kidney disease.

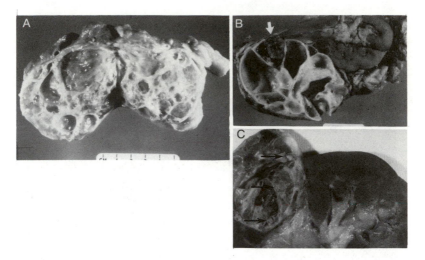

FIG 2–55.
Multilocular cyst versus cystic RCC. **A,** gross photograph of excised mass that proved to be a multilocular renal cyst. **B,** loculated cystic mass with solid RCC growing in the wall of one of the loculated cysts (*white arrow*). **C,** loculated cystic mass similar in appearance to multilocular cyst, but three areas of definite RCC were identified in the walls of the cysts (*black arrows*). Preoperative confirmation of diagnosis would be extremely difficult.

of flattened to hobnailed cells with fibrous septa separating the cysts and with demarcation from the normal parenchyma by a fibrous capsule.[49]

Renal Medullary Interstitial Tumor.—Formerly termed a *medullary fibroma,* the renal medullary interstitial tumor is a common small tan nodule (<1 cm) in renal medullary tissue. Multiple lesions may be present. It is important to recognize these entities and not to confuse them with small satellite nodules of an RCC or multiple adenomas. They are rarely identified preoperatively and are clinically insignificant. Microscopic examination identifies a fibrous tumor with collagen, scattered spindle cells, entrapped tubules, and indistinct margins.[48, 49]

Hemangioma and Lymphangioma.—Hemangiomas and lymphangiomas are benign neoplasms arising from blood vessels and lymph vessels, respectively.[48, 49] Both are rare and generally present clinically with hematuria; no characteristic imaging patterns are evident, and they are generally hypervascular on angiography. Hemangiomas are usually small (1 to 2 cm) solid lesions in the kidney, and complete excisional biopsy of the mass is reasonable. Lymphangiomas are larger tumors and probably require a nephrectomy for diagnosis, as preoperative differentiation from the more common RCC would be difficult.

Juxtaglomerular Cell Tumor.—A juxtaglomerular cell tumor is an extremely rare benign lesion arising from smooth muscle of the afferent arteriole and is characterized by renin production, which is relieved by resection of the tumor.[94] It is believed to be a specialized form of hemangiopericytoma. The tumors are usually tan, small, typically seen in younger individuals than those with RCC, and have associated substantial diastolic hypertension. Imaging studies indicate a solid, vascular mass. Several cases of renin-producing RCC have also been reported,[44] but histologic differentiation between these two lesions has been possible.[95]

Capsular and Perirenal Lesions.—Mass lesions of varying size, often symptomatic because of their large size, may arise from a multitude of mesenchymal cells ultimately leading to the development of a lipoma, leiomyoma, or fibroma.[96] Because these lesions are slow growing, they can become large, with or without malignant degeneration. Histologic appearance is similar to that seen in other organs, and the microscopic differential from RCC is usually not problematic.[49] With the exception of the lipoma, which has a characteristic low density on CT scan, preoperative confirmation of the benign nature of the lesion is difficult. Angiographically the lesions are hypovascular but can occasionally have areas of abnormal vasculature.

II. Malignant Tumors

It is not uncommon that renal or retroperitoneal tumors can be identified preoperatively as malignant but that the exact histologic classification is not feasible until the entire specimen is removed. It behooves the clinician, however, to remember that these non-RCC malignancies may exist because occasionally preoperative or nonoperative therapy should be considered, special studies should be obtained on the specimen, or appropriate consultation should be obtained. A perfect example of this is renal lymphoma.

Lymphoproliferative Malignancies.—Isolated renal lymphoma is uncommon. Clinical features that might raise the possibility of a lymphoma and include bilateral masses, bulky retroperitoneal adenopathy, loss of planes around the kidney on imaging studies, and abnormal vasculature in the tumor without the typical arteriovenous shunting (Fig 2–56).[97, 98] None of these findings is specific but may raise the level of suspicion so that an aspiration or needle biopsy would be performed. Preoperative or intraoperative identification of the lymphoma is important to avoid what could be an ill-advised nephrectomy and to ensure that the pathologist receives adequate tissue samples in suitable condition to perform immunohistochemistry, immunocytometry, and genotyping. Often this can only be done on fresh frozen tissue or fresh cell suspensions.[99]

Microscopically the presence of large numbers of similar-appearing malignant cells within the interstitial tissue with compression and occasional sparing of glomeruli and tubules is an important clue to diagnosis (Fig 2–57).

Other lymphoproliferative diseases such as leukemia or multiple myeloma can involve the kidney. Isolated involvement is possible but extremely rare.[48] The cells in lymphoproliferative malignant tumors resemble those in lesions elsewhere in the body.

Epithelial Tumors of the Pelvis.—Occasionally a large and high grade epithelial tumor of the renal pelvis, primarily a transitional cell carcinoma but also squamous cell carcinoma can invade the substance of the kidney and appear more as a mass lesion than the more typical filling defect in the collecting system. Recognition of this entity is important to ensure complete removal of the ureter at the time of nephrectomy and to dictate the need for cystoscopy

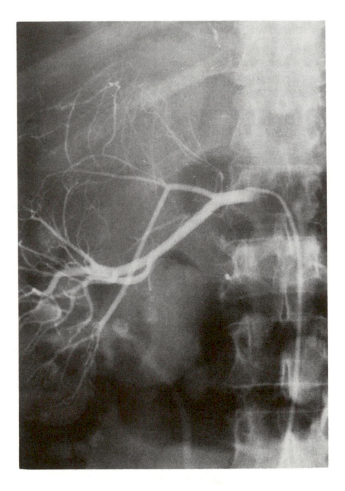

FIG 2–56.
Renal lymphoma. Arteriogram demonstrates hypovascular mass in the upper pole of the right kidney, which subsequently proved to be a renal lymphoma.

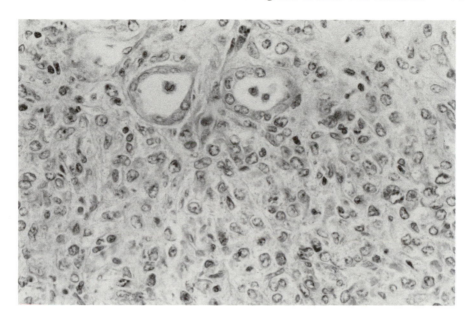

FIG 2–57.
Large cell non-Hodgkin's lymphoma. Numerous lymphoma cells with pleomorphic nuclei and isolated renal tubules. (Hematoxylin-eosin stain, magnification ×422.)

and optimal therapy. Transitional and squamous cell carcinomas demonstrate encasement of small renal vessels rather than typical arteriovenous shunting seen with RCC. Transitional cell carcinoma in this setting would likely be associated with positive results on a urine cytologic examination, whereas this finding is uncommon with RCC.

Adult Wilms' Tumor.—Although rare, the adult Wilms' tumor is a well defined entity that must be recognized. It is often a dilemma for a pathologist to differentiate between an RCC and renal sarcoma; it is important since adult Wilms' tumors are sensitive to chemotherapy and radiation therapy as are the tumors in children.[100] The tumor is generally seen in young adults and is symptomatic. Recognition of the primitive blastema, stroma, and the presence of abortive or embryonic glomeruli and/or tubular structures without any glandular elements seen in RCC are needed to establish the diagnosis.[48, 49] Preoperative imaging studies are not different from RCC, but the younger age of the patient should raise some suspicion of the diagnosis (Fig 2–58).

Metastatic Carcinoma of the Kidney.—Bracken et al[101] has stated that secondary carcinomas of the kidneys are more common than primary tumors based on an incidence of 7% renal involvement in an autopsy study of 11,000 cases of patients dying of malignant disease. Because of improved abdominal imaging studies, we now identify these lesions commonly, and occasionally they are symptomatic and require treatment (Fig 2–59). Clues that cause one to entertain this diagnosis are the obvious existence of the initial carcinoma in another organ and hypovascularity of the renal tumor. Aspiration or needle biopsy of the renal tumor can be helpful and may obviate an ill-advised operation. The metastases to the kidney are bilateral in approximately 50% of cases, and the most common sites of the primary tumor are lung, melanoma, breast, gastrointestinal tract, and genitourinary tract (Fig 2–60).

Adrenocortical Carcinoma.—In patients with large tumors in the region of the upper pole of a kidney, it may be impossible to differentiate clinically between an RCC and an adrenocortical carcinoma (Fig 2–61).[48] Adrenal tumors are less common, may be functionally active with signs of steroid excess, and usually compress the upper pole of the kidney without invading it. Pathologic distinction is important because palliation can be done with systemic therapy for adrenocortical carcinoma; however, the histologic differentiation can also be quite difficult (Fig 2–62). Distinction between the tumors depends on finding typical histologic patterns of RCC. A small biopsy specimen of an anaplastic tumor may be difficult to interpret. RCC cells may contain glycogen. Cells of both tumors may contain lipid.

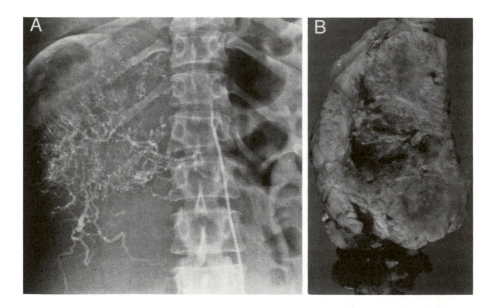

FIG 2–58.
Adult Wilms' tumor. **A,** arteriographic phase of large right upper quadrant mass shows marked parasitization of abnormal blood vessels. Remnant of parenchyma is present in upper pole. **B,** gross photograph of specimen shows marked "fleshy" appearance of the tumor.

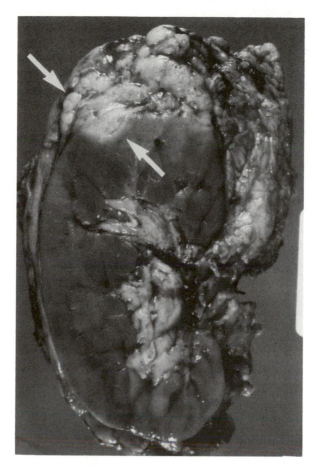

FIG 2–59.
Metastatic carcinoma to the kidney with invasion of the upper pole and perinephric soft tissue (*white arrows*).

Sarcomas.—As is the case with benign mesenchymal lesions, liposarcoma, leiomyosarcoma, fibrosarcomas, and malignant fibrous histiocytomas can occur in kidney or perirenal tissue (Fig 2–63).[102] Characterized by their large size and relative hypovascularity, there is quite frequent local extension, and resection can be difficult. For well-differentiated lesions, a subtotal excision can be worthwhile because of an indolent growth rate, but usually the prognosis is poor. Soft tissue sarcomas are usually treated with chemotherapy and radiation therapy based on the histologic type of the tumor.

Malignant fibrous histiocytoma is an increasingly recognized malignancy in several areas of the body, including the kidney and retroperitoneum. The sarcoma has a spindle cell pattern, is usually symptomatic and large at presentation, is difficult to remove surgically, and is associated with a poor prognosis (Fig 2–64).[49, 103]

A hemangiopericytoma is a particular type of soft tissue tumor characterized by a proliferation of spindle cells around endothelial-lined channels.[49, 104] These tumors may behave in a benign or malignant pattern. They are commonly richly vascular, large, and cystic, and venous invasion has been reported. The ultrastructural pattern is characteristic based on the origin of the tumor from pericytes.

Renal Cell Carcinoma Metastases to Other Organs

Because RCC can have symptoms from identifiable metastases, some discussion is appropriate relative to particular characteristics of these metastases. Approximately 30% of patients with RCC have metastases at the time of diagnosis, and 10% have symptoms secondary to these metastases. Several situations should be discussed either because of their frequency or because of problems associated with establishing a diagnosis.[48]

Lung metastases are extremely common in RCC (Fig 2–65). A potential area of confusion can arise with a benign clear cell tumor of the lung. Histochemical and ultrastructural studies can differentiate between the two.[105] Clear cell RCC usually has a characteristic vascular pattern.

Liver metastases are highly vascular solid lesions that must be differentiated clinically from the common benign hemangioma. Bone metastases usually are

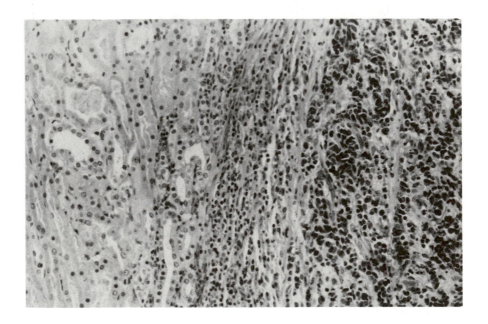

FIG 2–60.
Metastatic small cell carcinoma of uterine cervix in kidney. Tumor cells contain somewhat oval hyperchromatic nuclei and little cytoplasm (*right*). Renal tubules are at *left*. (Hematoxylin-eosin stain, magnification ×206.)

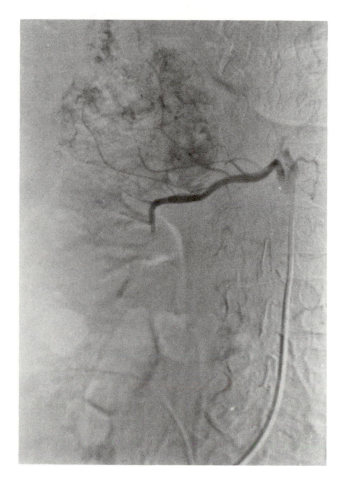

FIG 2–61.
Adrenocortical carcinoma. IV digital subtraction angiography demonstrates hypervascular upper pole mass in the right kidney. Angiographically it would not be possible to differentiate this lesion from a primary RCC.

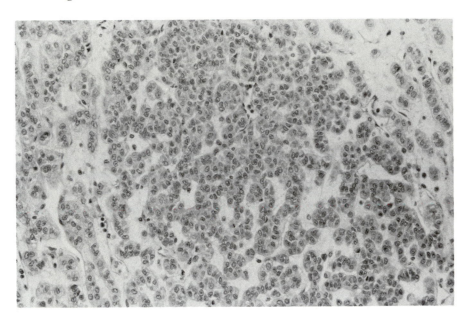

FIG 2–62.
Adrenocortical carcinoma. Trabeculae of tumor cells with irregular nuclei, granular, and occasionally vacuolated cytoplasm. (Hematoxylin-eosin stain, magnification ×206.)

symptomatic and are frequently in the proximal long bones, shoulder girdle, or pelvis. An orthopedic surgeon operating on this lytic lesion may encounter extreme bleeding from these richly vascular tumors (Fig 2–66).

Central nervous system lesions may pose problems secondary to histologic similarities between a primary hemangioblastoma of the brain (often seen with von Hippel-Lindau disease, as is RCC). Skin metastases can be confused with sebaceous carcinoma or nodular hidradenoma. Ovarian metastases can be confused with clear cell carcinoma of the ovary; salivary gland metastases and thyroid metastases can also be confused with primary tumors in the organs (Fig 2–67).

RCC can and does metastasize almost anywhere, and case reports of bizarre presentations abound.[49] The first clue to the clinician may be the inordinate bleeding encountered at the time of biopsy or resection. The histologic pattern may further suggest the renal origin, thus leading to appropriate imaging studies. Some metastatic RCCs may not have the usual clear cell or granular cell morphology. In cases with a sarcomatoid appearance the pathologist should consider the kidney as a possible site of origin.

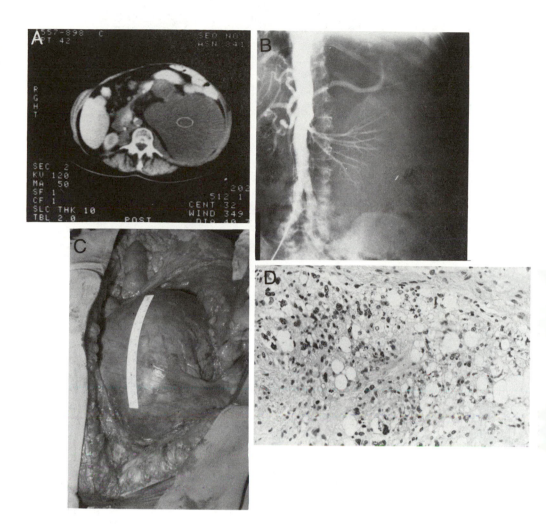

FIG 2–63.
Liposarcoma. **A,** CT demonstrates soft tissue mass in right abdomen displacing kidney. This patient had previous local excisions of retroperitoneal lipoma. **B,** arteriogram demonstrates encasement of renal vessels by large tumor mass that is relatively hypovascular. **C,** gross photograph of 25 cm liposarcoma involving right retroperitoneum and kidney. **D,** perirenal liposarcoma. Lobules of lipoblasts with variable nuclear size, shape, and chromaticity. Trabeculated cytoplasm contains lipid. (Hematoxylin-eosin stain, magnification ×206.)

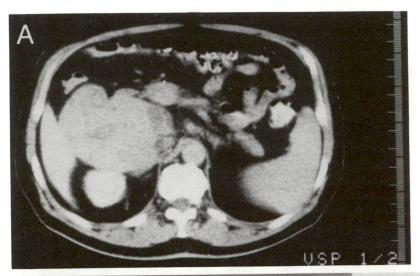

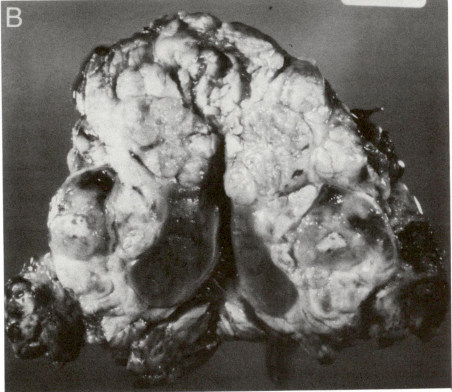

FIG 2–64.
Malignant fibrous histiocytoma. **A,** CT demonstrates retroperitoneal tumor encasing and invading IVC. **B,** lesion invading and replacing renal parenchyma.

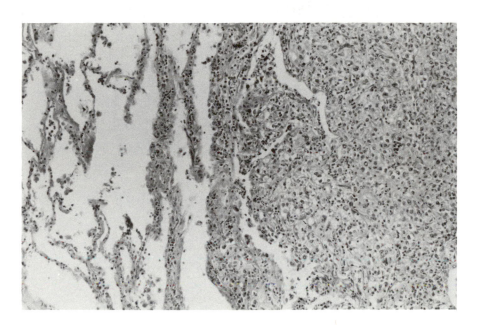

FIG 2–65.
Metastatic granular cell RCC in lung. (Hematoxylin-eosin stain, magnification ×103.)

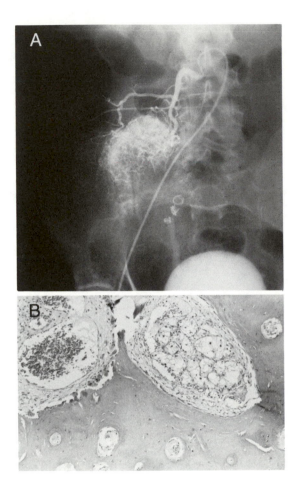

FIG 2–66.
A, angiogram demonstrates typical extreme hypervascularity of metastatic lesion in right side of pelvic bone. **B,** metastatic RCC in bone. Adjacent bone shows osteoclastic activity (*left*). (Hematoxylin-eosin stain, magnification ×103.)

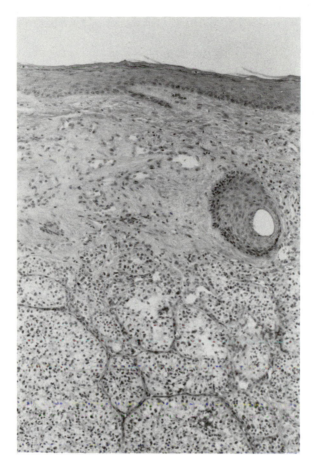

FIG 2–67.
Scalp. Nest of metastatic RCC in dermis. (Hematoxylin-eosin stain, magnification × 103.)

REFERENCES

1. Kiely JM: Hypernephroma—The internist's tumor. *Med Clin North Am* 1966; 50:1067–1083.
2. Gibbons RP, Montie JE, Correa RJ, et al: Manifestations of renal cell carcinoma. *Urology* 1976; 8:201–206.
3. Sogani PC, Whitmore WF: Solitary vaginal metastasis from unsuspected renal cell carcinoma. *J Urol* 1979; 121:95–97.
4. Burt ME, Brenan MF: Incidence of hypercalcemia and malignant neoplasm. *Arch Surg* 1980; 115:704–707.
5. Broadus AE, Mangin M, Ikeda K, et al: Humoral hypercalcemia of cancer. *N Engl J Med* 1988; 319:556–562.
6. Brereton HD, Halushka PV, Alexander RW, et al: Indomethacin-responsive hypercalcemia in a patient with renal-cell adenocarcinoma. *N Engl J Med* 1974; 291:83–85.
7. Aoki J, Yamamoto I, Hino M, et al: Osteoclast-mediated osteolysis in bone metastasis from renal cell carcinoma. *Cancer* 1988; 62:98–104.
8. Altaffer LF, Chenault OW: Paraneoplastic endocrinopathies associated with renal tumors. *J Urol* 1979; 122:573–577.
9. Pavelic K, Popovici M: Insulin and glucagon secretion by renal adenocarcinoma. *Cancer* 1981; 48:98–100.
10. Mukamel E, Nissenkorn I, Avidor I, et al: Spontaneous rupture of renal and ureteral tumors presenting as acute abdominal condition. *J Urol* 1979; 122:696–698.
11. Fletcher MS, Packham DA, Pryor JP, et al: Hepatic dysfunction in renal carcinoma. *Br J Urol* 1981; 53:533–536.
12. Stauffer MH: Nephrogenic hepatosplenomegaly (abstract). *Gastroenterology* 1961; 40:694.
13. Loughlin KR, Gittes RF, Partridge D, et al: The relationship of lactoferrin to the anemia of renal cell carcinoma. *Cancer* 1987; 59:566–571.
14. von Knorring J, Selroos O, Scheinin TM: Haematologic findings in patients with renal carcinoma. *Scand J Urol Nephrol* 1981; 15:279–283.
15. Nseyo UO, Williams PD, Murphy GP: Clinical significance of erythropoietin levels in renal carcinoma. *Urology* 1986; 28:301–306.
16. Sytkowski AJ, Bicknell KA, Smith GM, et al: Secretion of erythropoietin-like activity by clones of human renal carcinoma of cell line GKA. *Cancer Res* 1984; 44:51–54.
17. Kutty K, Varkey B: Incidence and distribution of intrathoracic metastases from renal cell carcinoma. *Arch Intern Med* 1984; 144:273–276.
18. Badlani G, Pillari G, Hajdu E, et al: Primary renal or pulmonary tumor—A diagnostic dilemma. *J Urol* 1981; 125:721–724.
19. Paul JG, Rhodes DB, Skow JR: Renal cell carcinoma presenting as right atrial tumor with successful removal using cardiopulmonary bypass. *Ann Surg* 1975; 181:471–473.
20. Melman A, Grim CE, Weinberger MH: Increased incidence of renal cell carcinoma with hypertension. *J Urol* 1977; 118:531–532.
21. Gay PC, Litchy WJ, Cascino TL: Brain metastasis in hypernephroma. *J Neurooncol* 1987; 5:51–56.
22. Sundaresan N, Scher H, DiGiacinto GV, et al: Surgical treatment of spinal cord compression in kidney cancer. *J Clin Oncol* 1986; 4:1851–1856.

23. Case records of the Massachusetts General Hospital (Case 1–1978). *N Engl J Med* 1978; 298:95–101.
24. Ritch PS, Hansen RM, Collier BD: Metastatic renal cell carcinoma presenting as shoulder arthritis. *Cancer* 1983; 51:968–972.
25. Case records of the Massachusetts General Hospital (Case 42–1980). *N Engl J Med* 1980; 303:985–995.
26. McDonald JR, Priestley JT: Malignant tumors of the kidney. *Surg Gynecol Obstet* 1943; 77:295–306.
27. Flocks RH, Kadesky MC: Malignant neoplasms of the kidney: An analysis of 353 patients followed five years or more. *J Urol* 1958; 79:196–201.
28. Robson CJ: Radical nephrectomy for renal cell carcinoma. *J Urol* 1963; 89:37–42.
29. Robson CJ, Churchill BM, Anderson W: The results of radical nephrectomy for renal cell carcinoma. *J Urol* 1969; 101:297–301.
30. Skinner DG, Colvin RB, Vermillion CD, et al: Diagnosis and management of renal cell carcinoma. *Cancer* 1971; 28:1165–1176.
31. Beahrs OH, Henson DE, Hutter RV, et al: *Manual for Staging of Cancer.* Philadelphia, JB Lippincott Company, 1987.
32. Siminovitch JMP, Montie JE, Straffon RA: Prognostic indicators in renal adenocarcinoma. *J Urol* 1983; 130:20–23.
33. Selli C, Hinshaw WM, Woodard BH, et al: Stratification of risk factors in renal cell carcinoma. *Cancer* 1983; 52:899–903.
34. Bassil B, Dosoretz DE, Prout GR: Validation of the tumor, nodes, and metastasis classification of renal cell carcinoma. *J Urol* 1985; 134:450–454.
35. Droller MJ: Renal cell carcinoma/oncocytoma, in Resnick MI, Caldamone AA, Sprinak JP (eds): *Decision Making in Urology.* Toronto, BC Decker, Inc, 1985, pp 92–93.
36. McClennan BL: Computed tomography in the diagnosis and staging of renal cell carcinoma. *Semin Urol* 1985; 3:111–131.
37. Davidson AJ, Hartman DS: Imaging strategies for tumors of the kidney, adrenal gland, and retroperitoneum. *CA* 1987; 37:151–164.
38. Friedland GW, Filly R, Goris ML, et al: *Uroradiology: An integraded approach.* New York, Churchill Livingstone, Inc, 1985.
39. Lang EK: Roentgenographic assessment of asymptomatic renal lesions. *Radiology* 1973; 109:257–269.
40. Brooks AP: Prostatism, intravenous urography and asymptomatic renal cancer. *Br J Urol* 1988; 62:1–3.
41. Dalton D, Neiman H, Grayhack JT: The natural history of simple renal cysts: A preliminary study. *J Urol* 1986; 135:905–908.
42. Frohmuller HGW, Grups JW, Heller V: Comparative value of ultrasonography, computerized tomography, angiography and excretory urography in the staging of renal cell carcinoma. *J Urol* 1987; 138:482–484.
43. Kam J, Sandler CM, Benson GS: Angiography in diagnosis of renal tumors. *Urology* 1981; 18:100–106.
44. Engelmann U, Schaub T, Schweden F, et al: Digital subtraction angiography in staging renal cell carcinoma: Comparison with computerized tomography and histopathology. *J Urol* 1984; 132:1093–1096.
45. Zabbo A, Novick AC, Risius B, et al: Digital subtraction angiography for evaluating patients with renal carcinoma. *J Urol* 1985; 134:252–255.

46. Siminovitch JMP, Montie JE, Straffon RA: Inferior venacavography in the preoperative assessment of renal adenocarcinoma. *J Urol* 1982; 128:908–909.
47. Feldman AE, Pollack HM, Perri AJ, et al: Renal pseudotumors: An anatomic-radiologic classification. *J Urol* 1978; 120:133–139.
48. Bennington JL, Beckwith JB: *Tumors of the Kidney, Renal Pelvis, and Ureter.* Washington, D.C., Armed Forces Institute of Pathology, 1975.
49. Petersen RO: *Urologic Pathology.* Philadelphia, JB Lippincott, Co, 1986.
50. Bell ET: A classification of renal tumors with observations on the frequency of the various types. *J Urol* 1938; 39:238.
51. Fuhrman SA, Lasky LC, Limas C: Prognostic significance of morphologic parameters in renal cell carcinoma. *Am J Surg Pathol* 1982; 6:655–663.
52. Thompson IM, Peek M: Improvement in survival of patients with renal cell carcinoma—The role of the serendipitously detected tumor. *J Urol* 1988; 140:487–490.
53. Kendall AR, Senay BA, Coll ME: Spontaneous subcapsular renal hematoma: Diagnosis and management. *J Urol* 1988; 139:246–250.
54. Mydlo JH, Bard RH: Analysis of papillary renal adenocarcinoma. *Urology* 1987; 30:529–534.
55. Marshall FF, Taxy JB, Fishman EK, et al: The feasibility of surgical enucleation for renal cell carcinoma. *J Urol* 1986; 135:231–234.
56. Blackley SK, Ladaga L, Woolfitt RA, et al: Ex situ study of the effectiveness of enucleation in patients with renal cell carcinoma. *J Urol* 1988; 140:6–10.
57. Patterson J, Lohr D, Briscoe C, et al: Calcified renal masses. *Urology* 1987; 29:353–356.
58. Daniel WW, Hartman GW, Witten DM, et al: Calcified renal masses. *Radiology* 1972; 103:503–508.
59. Johnson CD, Dunnick NR, Cohan RH, et al: Renal adenocarcinoma: CT staging of 100 tumors. *AJR* 1987; 148:59–63.
60. Giuliani L, Giberti C, Martorana G, et al: Value of computerized tomography and ultrasonography in the preoperative diagnosis of renal cell carcinoma extending into the inferior vena cava. *Eur Urol* 1987; 13:26–30.
61. Pritchett TR, Ravol JK, Benson RC, et al: Preoperative magnetic resonance imaging of vena caval thrombi: Experience with 5 cases. *J Urol* 1987; 138:1220–1222.
62. Pizzocaro G, Piva L, Salvioni R: Lymph node dissection in radical nephrectomy for renal cell carcinoma: Is it necessary? *Eur Urol* 1983; 9:10–12.
63. Marshall FF, Powell KC: Lymphadenectomy for renal cell carcinoma: Anatomical and therapeutic considerations. *J Urol* 1982; 128:677–680.
64. Siminovitch JP, Montie JE, Straffon RA: Lymphadenectomy in renal adenocarcinoma. *J Urol* 1982; 127:1090–1091.
65. Herrlinger A, Schrott KM, Siege A, et al: Results of 381 transabdominal radical nephrectomies for renal cell carcinoma with partial and complete en-bloc lymph-node dissection. *World J Urol* 1984; 2:114–121.
66. Robey EL, Schellhammer PF: The adrenal gland and renal cell carcinoma: Is ipsilateral adrenalectomy a necessary component of radical nephrectomy? *J Urol* 1986; 135:453–455.
67. Reis M, Faria V: Renal carcinoma: Reevaluation of prognostic factors. *Cancer* 1988; 61:1192–1199.
68. Medeiros LJ, Gelb AB, Weiss LM: Renal cell carcinoma: Prognostic significance of morphologic parameters in 121 cases. *Cancer* 1988; 61:1639–1651.

69. Tomera KM, Farrow GM, Lieber MM: Sarcomatoid renal carcinoma. *J Urol* 1983; 130:657–659.

70. Bonsib SM, Fischer J, Plattner S, et al: Sarcomatoid renal tumors: Clinicopathologic correlation of three cases. *Cancer* 1987; 59:527–532.

71. Shirkhoda A, Lewis E: Renal sarcoma and sarcomatoid renal cell carcinoma: CT and angiographic features. *Radiology* 1987; 162:353–357.

72. Tomera KM, Farrow GM, Lieber MM: Well differentiated (grade 1) clear cell renal carcinoma. *J Urol* 1983; 129:933–937.

73. Press GA, McClennan BL, Melson GL, et al: Papillary renal cell carcinoma: CT and sonographic evaluation. *AJR* 1984; 143:1005–1009.

74. Selli C, Hinshaw WM, Woodard BH, et al: Stratification of risk factors in renal cell carcinoma. *Cancer* 1983; 52:899–903.

75. Carroll PR, Murty VVS, Reuter V, et al: Abnormalities at chromosome region 3p12–14 characterize clear cell renal carcinoma. *Cancer Genet Cytogenet* 1987; 26:253–259.

76. Zbar B, Brouch H, Talmadge C, et al: Loss of alleles of loci on the short arm of chromosome 3 in renal cell carcinoma. *Nature* 1987; 327:721.

77. Bander NH: Comparison of antigen expression of human renal cancers in vivo and in vitro. *Cancer* 1984; 53:1235–1239.

78. Bander NH: Monoclonal antibodies: State of the art. *J Urol* 1987; 137:603–612.

79. Chiou RK, Vessella RL, Limas C: Monoclonal antibody-targeted radiotherapy of renal cell carcinoma using a nude mouse model. *Cancer* 1988; 61:1766–1775.

80. Ljungberg B, Forsslund G, Stenling R, et al: Prognostic significance of the DNA content in renal cell carcinoma. *J Urol* 1986; 135:422–426.

81. Yoshida MA, Ohyashiki K, Ochi H, et al: Cytogenetic studies of tumor tissue from patients with nonfamilial renal cell carcinoma. *Cancer Res* 1986; 46:2139–2147.

82. Mukamel E, Konichezky M, Engelstein D, et al: Incidental small renal tumors accompanying clinically overt renal cell carcinoma. *J Urol* 1988; 140:22–24.

83. Mostofi FK, Davis CJ: *Tumors and Tumor-Like Lesions of the Kidney.* Chicago, Year Book Medical Publishers, Inc, 1986.

84. Lieber MM, Tomera KM, Farrow GM: Renal oncocytoma. *J Urol* 1981; 125:481–485.

85. Maatman TJ, Novick AC, Tancinco BF, et al: Renal oncocytoma: A diagnostic and therapeutic dilemma. *J Urol* 1984; 132:878–881.

86. Psihramis KE, Cin PD, Dretler SP, et al: Further evidence that renal oncocytoma has malignant potential. *J Urol* 1988; 139:585–587.

87. Stillwell TJ, Gomez MR, Kelalis PP: Renal lesions in tuberous sclerosis. *J Urol* 1987; 138:477–481.

88. Blute ML, Malek RS, Segura JW: Angiomyolipoma: Clinical metamorphosis and concepts for management. *J Urol* 1988; 139:20–24.

89. Malek RS, Greene LF, DeWeerd JH, et al: Xanthogranulomatous pyelonephritis. *Br J Urol* 1972; 44:296–308.

90. Stanton MJ, Maxted W: Malacoplakia: A study of the literature and current concepts of pathogenesis, diagnosis and treatment. *J Urol* 1981; 125:139–146.

91. Spencer WC, Novick AC, Montie JE, et al: The surgical treatment of localized renal cell carcinoma in von Hippel-Lindau disease. *J Urol* 1988; 139:507–509.

92. Boileau M, Foley R, Flechner S, et al: Renal adenocarcinoma and end-stage kidney disease. *J Urol* 1987; 138:603–606.

93. Bretan PN, Busch MP, Hricak H, et al: Chronic renal failure: A significant risk factor in the development of acquired renal cysts and renal cell carcinoma. *Cancer* 1986; 57:1871–1879.

94. Squires JP, Ulbright TM, DeSchryver-Kecskemeti K, et al: Juxtaglomerular cell tumor of the kidney. *Cancer* 1984; 53:516–523.
95. Lindop GBM, Leckie B, Winearls CG: Malignant hypertension due to a renin-secreting renal cell carcinoma—An ultrastructural and immunocytochemical study. *Histopathology* 1986; 10:1077–1088.
96. Myerson D, Rosenfield AT, Itzchak Y: Renal capsular tumors: The angiographic features. *J Urol* 1979; 121:238–241.
97. Siegel SW, Risius B, Tubbs R, et al: Bilateral solid renal masses in a young man. *J Urol* 1986; 135:327–330.
98. Osborne BM, Brenner M, Weitzner S, et al: Malignant lymphoma presenting as a renal mass: Four cases. *Am J Surg Pathol* 1987; 11:375–382.
99. Pontes JE, Tubbs RR: Lymphoproliferative disorders. *J Urol* 1987; 137:958.
100. Chung TS, Reyes CV, Stefani SS: Wilms tumor in adults. *Urology* 1984; 24:275–277.
101. Bracken RB, Chica G, Johnson DE, et al: Secondary renal neoplasms: An autopsy study. *South Med J* 1979; 72:806–807.
102. Srinivas V, Sogani PC, Hajdu SI, et al: Sarcomas of the kidney. *J Urol* 1984; 132:13–16.
103. Ojeda LM, Johnson DE, Ames FC, et al: Primary renal malignant fibrous histiocytoma. *Urology* 1984; 24:491–494.
104. Ordonez NG, Bracken RB, Stroehlein KB: Hemangiopericytoma of kidney. *Urology* 1982; 20:191–195.
105. Carter D, Eggleston JC: Tumors of the lower respiratory tract. Washington, D.C., Armed Forces Institute of Pathology, 1979, p, 920.

Part *II*

Surgical Aspects

3

Radical Nephrectomy, Lymphadenectomy, and Local Adjuvant Therapies

J. Edson Pontes, M.D.

RADICAL NEPHRECTOMY

Radical nephrectomy is presently the accepted method of initial treatment for patients with localized renal cell carcinoma (RCC). Because no other modalities of therapy are available for the treatment of this malignancy, surgery continues to be the only option available. The technical aspects of performance of this operation are well known and are discussed only generally in this chapter. We do discuss, however, several issues that led to the widespread use of this procedure as opposed to simple nephrectomy, such as its influence on survival and the decrease of local recurrence. In the next two sections issues closely related to radical nephrectomy such as the value of lymphadenectomy and the place of adjunctive methods such as radiation therapy and angioinfarction are discussed.

Technical Aspects of Radical Nephrectomy

The surgical approach for radical nephrectomy varies according to individual choice and to technical problems associated with tumor location, size, etc. Most surgeons use the anterior rather than the flank approach. The transabdominal approach with either a longitudinal midline or transverse Chevron incision approach are the most popular.[1] Alternatives are the thoracoabdominal incision used mainly for upper pole or large tumors (Fig 3–1). In all these approaches the goals are early access to the renal pedicle to avoid manipulation of the tumor and dissemination, removal en bloc of Gerota's fascia and peri-

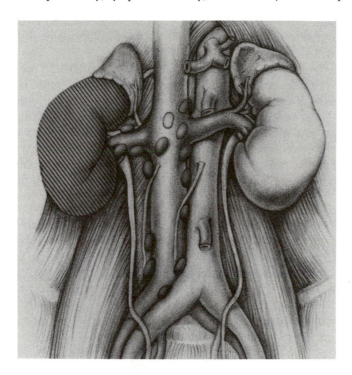

FIG 3–1.
Lymph node drainage from the right kidney. (Modified from Marshall FF, Powell KC: *J Urol* 1982; 128:677, and Pizzocaro G: Lymphadenectomy in renal adenocarcinoma, in deKernion JB, Pavone-Macaluso M (eds): *Tumors of the Kidney.* Baltimore, Williams & Wilkins, 1986, p 75.)

nephric fat, and excision of perihilar nodes.[1] Figures 3–2 and 3–3 show the surgical approach to the renal pedicle on the right and left.

Critical Analysis of Factors Favoring Radical Nephrectomy

Several factors have been identified and proposed as possible benefits for radical nephrectomy such as early ligation of the renal pedicle to prevent tumor manipulation and dissemination and wider excision of perinephric fat and Gerota's fascia to decrease local recurrence.

The concept of early ligation of the pedicle to prevent dissemination from tumor manipulation (nontouch technique), popularized in surgical oncology, is now widely used. Although the idea is reasonable, biologically after a tumor reaches a size that is recognized clinically, there is a constant escape of tumor cells into the circulation.[2] Despite this, only a small percentage of patients will develop metastasis as a result of the inefficiency of the metastatic process.[3]

The concept of wider excision, including the perinephric fat and Gerota's fascia, was introduced after the observation by Beare and McDonald[4] showing a high percentage of patients with microscopic involvement of the capsule and the perinephric tissue. This observation led to the development of radical excision initially proposed by Chute et al,[5] Foley et al,[6] and later popularized by Robson et al.[7]

Despite the fact that anatomically this idea is sound, there has never been a prospective study comparing radical nephrectomy with simple nephrectomy. Therefore most of the advantages of this technique are based on historical data. Most of the arguments used today in favor of radical nephrectomy are based on the improved survival obtained by Robson et al.[7] Although there was a substantial improvement in survival in that series,[7] as compared with earlier ones, better patient selection with extensive metastatic workups, which included mediastinoscopy, probably played a role in the improvement of the results.

Results of Treatment and Impact of Radical Nephrectomy on Survival

In analyzing the results of the treatment of RCC at the Massachusetts General Hospital, Boston, Skinner et al[8] reviewed 309 cases that involved operations between 1935 and 1965. Of these, 93 patients had simple nephrectomies between

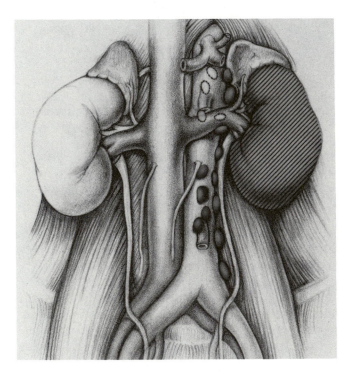

FIG 3–2.
Lymph node drainage from the left kidney. (Modified from Marshall FF, Powell KC: *J Urol* 1982; 128:677, and Pizzocaro G: Lymphadenectomy in renal adenocarcinoma, in deKernion JB, Pavone-Macaluso M (eds): *Tumors of the Kidney.* Baltimore, Williams & Wilkins, 1986, p 75.)

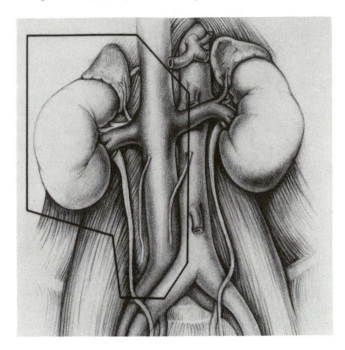

FIG 3–3.
Proposed limits of lymph node dissection of right kidney. (Modified from Marshall FF, Powell KC: *J Urol* 1982; 128:677, and Pizzocaro G: Lymphadenectomy in renal adenocarcinoma, in deKernion JB, Pavone-Macaluso M (eds): *Tumors of the Kidney.* Baltimore, Williams & Wilkins, 1986, p 75.)

1935 and 1948, whereas 203 patients had radical nephrectomies.[8] Analysis of the data by stage demonstrated no significant difference in survival. They[8] noted, however, that a firm conclusion could not be established, since patient selection and ability of the surgeon often dictated the form of treatment. Fifty-two percent of simple nephrectomies were performed for stage I, whereas only 24% of radical nephrectomies were done for tumors in this low stage. There was certainly a tendency to exclude from a surgical series patients with more extensive tumors that probably were considered inoperable and were therefore excluded from analysis. The differences in survival between simple nephrectomy and radical nephrectomy are particularly striking when comparisons are made with old published series. Skinner et al[8] cited that the earlier experience at the Massachusetts General Hospital, published by Mintz and Gaul[9] showed that among patients who had operations from 1900 to 1935, the 5-year survival was only 13%. In reviewing 235 simple nephrectomies performed at the New York Hospital—Cornell Medical Center, New York City, between 1932 and 1952, Humphreys and Foot[10] showed that approximately 50% of patients died at 3 years.

Robson et al[7] compared his series in 1969 with reports by Priestley,[11] Kaufman and Mims,[12] and Mostofi[13] and showed a significant improvement in survival. He attributed his success to early ligation of the pedicle with prevention of tumor emboli, wide excision of perinephric fat and Gerota's fascia, and extensive lymph node dissection. Middleton and Presto[14] compared their results in 61 patients who had operations by radical thoracoabdominal nephrectomy between 1950 and 1967 with those of Humphreys and Foot[10] who had operations at the same institution between 1932 and 1952 by simple nephrectomy. They showed a significant improvement in survival in the latter series.

Patel and Lavengood[15] reviewed 166 cases of patients treated at their institution between 1939 and 1977. Of these, 85 patients underwent simple nephrectomy, whereas the remaining had a radical approach. In their series[15] there was a significant improvement in survival for the latter.

Because of a lack of prospective comparative studies, it is impossible to objectively determine the impact of radical nephrectomy on survival. Factors that influence such an analysis are better selection of patients because of more sophisticated medical technology, better postoperative care on one hand and on the other hand the tendency to perform surgery in more advanced cases on the basis of improved surgical skills.[8]

The influence of local recurrence in the treatment of RCC is difficult to analyze. On the basis of the fact that a significant percentage of patients will have microscopic involvement of the capsule and perinephric fat, it is reasonable to assume that radical nephrectomy will decrease local recurrence. Analysis of the majority of series on radical nephrectomy failed to address this problem. This is most likely related to the fact that most patients who would develop local recurrence because of the extent of their tumor are also most likely to develop distant metastasis. In only one series[16] was the comparison of survival of patients with metastatic disease made with those patients with or without local recurrence. In that study there was a slight advantage in survival of patients without local recurrence. The number of patients, however, was small, and the persistence of tumor after operation was included with local recurrence.[16] The fact that a complete lymphadenectomy is not done in most series further confuses the issue, since some of the "local" recurrence may be the result of metastatic lymph nodes.

In summary, radical nephrectomy continues to be the accepted, standard treatment for localized RCC. Despite the fact that no objective studies exist to prove an advantage of this procedure as compared with simple nephrectomy, the surgical principles and pathologic data available suggest that this is the procedure of choice in localized RCC.

LYMPHADENECTOMY

The role of lymphadenectomy in association with radical nephrectomy in patients with RCC is controversial. The debate focuses initially on the anatomy of the renal lymphatic vessels and on the boundaries of dissection. Furthermore, the value of this procedure in a disease that shows early vascular invasion and metastasizes in an unpredictable manner has caused its effectiveness to be questioned. Besides the fact that lymphadenectomy is used in most malignancies as a staging procedure, in RCC the problem is compounded by the lack of a large clinical series that utilized lymphadenectomy in a standard manner. A review of the medical literature is therefore left to interpreting retrospective data that are often diverse, even in the same institution.

Lymphatic Drainage of the Kidney

The importance of a lymphatic system in the kidney has been documented by several authors.[17–19] Lymphatic capillary vessels provide a main function of draining the interstitium. A substantial amount of work demonstrating the concentration of electrolytes, glucose, and other "test" substances in the renal lymphatic system has been conducted by many investigators.[18, 20, 21]

Lymphatic output in the dog is approximately half that of urine.[18] With obstruction there is a significant increase of lymphatic output.[18] Connections between lymphatic and venous systems have been demonstrated.[22]

A study of the renal lymphatic vessels discloses two systems, one draining the medullary-cortical junction, exiting the kidney through six to eight channels at the hilum and another draining the cortical region, leaving by means of four to six channels in the renal capsule. Despite the observation that the hilum lymphatic vessels drain to lymph nodes of the hilar region, some lymphatic trunks drain directly into the thoracic duct.[18] Anatomic studies done by Parker[17] in 1935 failed to address these physiologic aspects, which were not known until the 1970s. Her studies,[17] however, established detailed information about the regional lymphatic vessels of the kidney.

In recent times the best description of the lymphatic drainage of the kidney comes from Marshall and Powell.[23] This has been confirmed by Pizzocaro.[24] According to these authors, the lymphatic drainage of the right kidney can be divided into anterior, middle, and posterior channels (see Figs 3–1 and 3–2). The anterior channels leave the kidney anterior to the renal vessels to end at the precaval nodes or curve upward to join the posterior lymphatic vessels.[23, 24] The posterior channels course superior and posterior to the renal vessels and drain into the postcaval and interaortic caval nodes from L1 to L3 and the upper lateral caval nodes. The middle lymphatic vessels course between the artery and the vein and join the posterior and anterior chains. Lymphatic channels can pass directly through the diaphragm to the thoracic duct. The left renal lymphatic vessels drain through anterior and posterior channels. These two groups of channels are drained into periaortic nodes with no substantial drainage to the interaortic caval area. The anterior group courses anterior to the renal vein with superior and inferior branches along the aorta occasionally interconnecting with the posterior group. The posterior group leaves the kidney posterior to the renal vessels and divides at the crus of the diaphragm into the superior and inferior branches. Superiorly they pass through the diaphragm and through the postaortic nodes between T11 and L1. Inferiorly they end at the left lateral lumbar nodes between the lower pole of the kidney and the renal vein. The regional nodes of the left kidney include the left lateral lumbar preaortic and postaortic nodes. Additional nodes are present in the crus of the diaphragm and at the left renal vein junction with the adrenal vein.[23, 24]

This detailed anatomic description forms the basis for modern lymphadenectomy as part of radical nephrectomy (Figs 3–3 and 3–4). There is, however, to my knowledge, no data available that correlate location of the tumor in the kidney with the predominance of one or other types of drainage or that reconcile the knowledge that channels leaving the renal hilum drain the corticomedullary region, and lymphatic vessels leaving through the renal capsule may drain primarily the cortical region.[18] How the location of a tumor or how invasion of the tumor capsule affects such drainage is presently unknown.

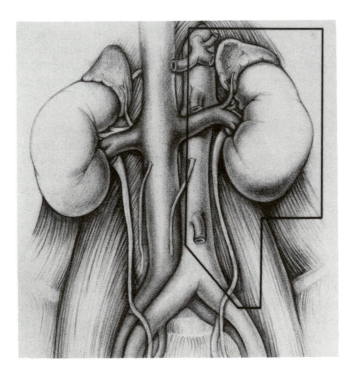

FIG 3–4.
Proposed limits of lymph node dissection of left kidney. (Modified from Marshall FF, Powell KC: *J Urol* 1982; 128:677, and Pizzocaro G: Lymphadenectomy in renal adenocarcinoma, in de-Kernion JB, Pavone-Macaluso M (eds): *Tumors of the Kidney.* Baltimore, Williams & Wilkins, 1986, p 75.)

TABLE 3–1.
Extended Lymphadenectomy in RCC

Author	Total % Positive	N + M$_0$ (%)	5-yr Survival for M$_0$ Patients (%)
Robson et al.[30]	22	NA	35
Giuliani et al.[31]	36	15 (15)	46
Hulten et al.[32]	27	NA	NA
Carl et al.[33]	23	133 (15)	NA
Sigel et al.[34]	29	NA	NA
Pizzocaro[24]	—	5	NA
Total	27%	15%	

N+ = positive nodes; M$_0$ = distant metastasis; NA = not applicable.

Lymphadenectomy in Renal Cell Carcinoma

Lymphadenectomy as part of radical nephrectomy has been performed on an individual basis with such a degree of variation that it would make standardization difficult. In this section I describe the extent of lymphadenectomy proposed by the authors who have done most of the work on identification of the lymphatic drainage of the kidney, and in the next section I discuss the available clinical data.

The concept of radical nephrectomy was popularized in the late 1940s and early 1950s based on the observation of detailed histologic studies that demonstrated that approximately 70% of patients had either invasion of the renal capsule or perinephric invasion.[25] The pioneers in proposing this procedure were Beare and McDonald,[25] Chute et al,[26] and Foley et al.[27] This operation took into account attempts in the beginning of the century at performing a more extensive procedure by many authors.[28, 29] With the exception of Chute, who described removal of the lymph nodes around the renal pedicle, little is discussed in relation to a formal lymphadenectomy. The series of Robson[30] in 1969 has served as a landmark for the use of radical nephrectomy because of the excellent results obtained. Despite the extent of the dissection performed in that series, however, lymphadenectomy was done "where possible" and included the paracaval nodes on the right and the paraaortic nodes on the left. In view of the present knowledge of the lymphatic drainage, this was clearly an incomplete node dissection.[23, 24]

A list of various series reported for radical nephrectomy with lymph node dissection is presented in Tables 3–1 and 3–2. In analyzing all series published on lymphadenectomy in RCC, it is clear that there are only a few studies that were done prospectively and only a few series in which a complete lymphadenectomy has been followed according to anatomic principles outlined earlier.

Specific information related to the number of patients without distant metastasis and the presence of positive nodes is sketchy. Often only a small number of patients are available for analysis, making statistical prediction unreliable. Among the series of patients undergoing extended lymph node dissection, some authors performed a dissection that included the interaortic caval nodes, retrocaval, and retroaortic.[23, 24, 31, 32] Despite extensive dissection, other authors[30] did not include these areas.

The extent of the regional node dissection is even more difficult to define. An overall analysis of all series published showed that approximately 27% of all patients undergoing extended node dissection had positive nodes as compared with 14% of those with regional dissection (see Tables 3–1 and 3–2). If an analysis is performed for patients without distant metastasis, the rates are 15% and 9%, respectively (see Table 3–1 and 3–2).

Analysis of Clinical Data

It is evident that the role of lymphadenectomy in surgery for RCC is difficult to define. Questions that need to be addressed include the extent of node dissection, morbidity associated with such a procedure, and the influence of node dissection on survival.

Because regionalization of lymphatic drainage as it relates to the location of the tumor in the kidney is not available, it will be impossible currently to make a rational recommendation for more limited dissection. Where do tumors that grow toward the hilum metastasize primarily? Do patients with T_1 tumors need extended dissection or just hilar nodal dissection? Should only patients with perinephric invasion have extended proposed dissection? Prospective studies that are carefully performed would answer such questions. The EORTC GU group is presently embarking on such a study.

The other factor associated with the decision of an extended node dissection

TABLE 3–2.
Regional Lymphadenectomy in RCC*

AUTHOR	TOTAL % POSITIVE	$N + M_0$ (%)	5-YR SURVIVAL FOR M_0 PATIENTS
Flocks and Kadesky[35]	25	21 (15)	14%
Rafla[36]	8	14 (7)	21%
Skinner et al.[42]	6	19 (8)	16%
Middleton and Presto[37]	11	7 (9)	—
Angervall and Wahlquist[38]	22	3 (9)	—
Waters and Richie[39]	24	8 (12)	—
Peters and Brown[40]	8	NA	—
Siminovitch et al.[41]	9	9 (9)	11%
Sigel[34]	14	—	—
Total	14%	9%	15%

*See Table 3–1 for explanation of abbreviations.

relates to the potential increase in morbidity that results from this operation. Although Robson et al[30] stated that the morbidity was not significantly increased with radical nephrectomy and extended node dissection, hospital mortality was 3.4%. Similarly Giuliani[31] noted that 10 patients died after surgery, although the cause of death was not discussed. Even with regional lymphadenectomy, most authors[42] report mortality around 4%. Some authors[24] therefore will not accept this increased morbidity for the potential small gain from this procedure.

The influence of node dissection on survival is extremely difficult to assess. If one analyzes the overall percentage of positive nodes in the absence of distant metastasis, there is a 6% difference among all series of patients in whom extended dissection or regional dissection was performed (15% versus 9%). The reason for this difference could be the result of a more extensive dissection, but it also could be simply a pathology artifact, since there is a tendency to "look" more if tissue location is specified, which probably was done more often in patients with extended dissection. Furthermore, the extent of regional dissection among different series was extremely variable, making any comparisons unreliable. If one analyzes the overall survival of patients with positive nodes in the absence of distant metastasis, it appears from published work that there is an advantage in patients undergoing extended dissection (see Tables 3–1 and 3–2). The numbers in individual series, however, are small, and the lack of information in large series makes any predictions unreliable.

It has been proposed that only 3% of all patients of the distant metastasis category will potentially benefit from a lymphadenectomy.[24] Other authors,[23] however, believe that as many as 5% to 10% of patients will benefit from this procedure. The question presently confronting us is that if there is a potential increase in morbidity and mortality for an extended lymphadenectomy, is there a justification for this procedure in view of the little benefit achieved.

ADJUVANT THERAPIES WITH SURGERY: THE ROLE OF RADIATION THERAPY AND ANGIOINFARCTION

Surgery has been the only known modality of treatment for RCC. In an attempt to improve the surgical results or to facilitate surgical removal of large tumors, other modalities of therapy have been tried in conjunction with nephrectomy. The two modalities most commonly used as adjunctive to surgical excision in RCC have been radiation therapy and angioinfarction.

Radiation Therapy

Radiotherapy in RCC has been used either as preoperative therapy in an attempt to facilitate surgery or as postoperative treatment to prevent local recurrence. The combination of radiation therapy and surgery was advocated about 40 to 50 years ago.[43, 44] Analysis of the series published in the 1950s suggested that radiation therapy had an influence in survival when associated with sur-

TABLE 3–3.
A Summary of Previous Series

REFERENCE	No. OF CASES	5-YR SURVIVAL FOR NEPHRECTOMY (%)	NEPHRECTOMY + RADIATION (%)
Flocks and Kadesky[46]	96	48	52
Richies et al.[47]	398	30	49
Peeling et al.[49]	164	52	25
Cox et al.[51]	100	44	32
Skinner et al.[52]	232	57	50
Finney[50]	105	44	36
Rafla[53]	190	37	56

gery.[45, 46] In 1966 Richies[47] reviewed his personal experience and indications for preoperative and postoperative radiation therapy for RCC and suggested that radiation therapy in either form improves survival in this population. In analyzing his series with postoperative radiation, he suggested that the value of this procedure was in patients with perinephric extension and lymphatic invasion. The indications for preoperative radiation therapy were proposed as decreasing the size of the tumor, decreasing the vascular supply, and making previously inoperable tumors operable.

A review[48] of large retrospective series of patients receiving adjunctive radiation therapy shows that the 5-year survival is not significantly improved. Only the study by Richies[47] suggested a significant benefit of radiation therapy at 5 years. Because of a slight improvement in survival in some series, cooperative studies were conducted in England by Peeling et al[49] and by Finney[50] that demonstrated no advantage of adjunctive radiation therapy to surgical tumor excision. A summary of previous series is shown in Table 3–3. Despite strong suggestive data that radiation therapy has no value in the treatment of RCC, some authors[51] have proposed specific angiographic and intraoperative changes to suggest a role in preoperative radiation therapy. Furthermore, some authors[54] have proposed the use of intraarterial chemotherapy plus radiation for large tumors in an attempt to decrease tumor size and improve operability.

Angioinfarction

Angioinfarction of primary RCC gained popularity in the 1970s after the description by Almgard et al,[55] suggesting that this procedure may increase operability of some lesions and may influence metastatic disease. The main goals of angioinfarction in RCC are improvement of surgical approach to large lesions by decreasing hemorrhage, making access to the renal pedicle easy and decreasing the size of the tumor; by palliative control of bleeding and pain in inoperable lesions; and by activation of some immunologic mechanisms by which metastatic lesions will stabilize or regress.[56] Several techniques have been utilized for producing angioinfarction. Since the description of Almgard et al,[55] who used autologous muscle mixed with contrast material, several other techniques have been proposed,[55, 57-61] including dextran autologous cloth, absorbable gelatin sponge (Gelfoam) and several types of coils, balloons, and more recently alcohol. Other more complicated procedures such as ferromagnetic infarction have not gained popularity.[62] The use of chemotherapeutic agents or radioactive seeds has been proposed for patients with inoperable lesions.[63] It is important to note that all those techniques are accompanied by postinfarction syndrome consisting of fever, pain, and ileus. There also have been complications associated such as accidental infarction of other organs with bowel necrosis, infarct of the opposite kidney, loss of a limb from dislodgment of a coil, and a spinal cord infarct.[56] I have observed a death in a patient who had a large caval thrombus, which after renal tumor embolization, produced a fatal pulmonary embolism.

It is important to note also that no matter which technique is used, infarction of the kidney is seldom complete, and with time revascularization of the tumor occurs. Surgically the two main advantages of angioinfarction are access to the renal pedicle in cases of medially located tumor, which makes the access to the renal artery difficult, and a decrease in intraoperative bleeding produced by the infarct. In the first instance there is no question that occlusion of the renal artery will allow ligation of the renal vein early, facilitating the procedure.

The decrease of intraoperative bleeding is less demonstrable because of the many variables present such as the type of case, the surgeon's ability, and other less objective factors. There are several studies[56] suggesting advantages of such a technique with a decrease of bleeding and operative time; however, there are others who see no advantage. I believe that there is a minority of highly selected patients in whom infarction preoperatively is of technical help.

The use of embolization of the primary tumor as a palliative therapy to decrease bleeding and pain has been proposed and discussed anecdotally by practicing physicians. There, however, are no large series illustrating its value. Because of the fact that angioinfarction is never complete, the benefits of such a procedure may be temporary. Finally, angioinfarction has been proposed by some[64] as a possible adjunct to nephrectomy in patients with metastatic disease. It has been proposed that some immunologic mechanism is activated by release of large quantities of tumor antigens that would trigger regression of some metastatic lesions and an increase in survival. Swanson et al[64] have shown in a few cases regression of pulmonary lesions and an increase of surviving patients treated at M. D. Anderson Hospital, Houston. We[65] have studied this problem in an experimental model and have been unable to demonstrate any improvement in immunologic activity after ischemia of a renal tumor.

Recently a prospective phase II study done by a cooperative group[66] showed no difference in response among patients treated with embolization in the presence of metastatic disease.

Adjunctive Treatment of Metastatic Lesions and the Role of Angioinfarction and Radiation Therapy

Metastasis of RCC to the bone is not uncommon. It has been suggested that approximately 50% of patients with metastatic RCC will eventually develop bony metastasis. In the presence of bony metastasis, treatment is mainly palliative to reduce pain and prevent pathologic fracture.

The use of angioinfarction for primary and metastatic lesions of the bones has been described by few authors.[67, 68] In our personal experience,[69] therapeutic embolization of large pelvic lytic metastasis offered significant local objective control of the lesions with partial calcification and a decrease in size in four of five patients treated. There was also significant subjective improvement with a decrease in pain and better performance status. The combination of embolization with chemotherapy or radioactive seeds has also been described with good local control.[63, 70]

Radiation therapy to metastatic RCC has long been used as palliation for pain, prevention of paraplegia in spinal cord lesions, or a decrease of mediastinal masses.[48] A decrease in bone pain and tumor size response have been reported in a significant percentage of patients.

REFERENCES

1. Montie JE: Management of stages I, II, and III renal adenocarcinoma, in Javadpour N (ed): *Principles and Management of Urologic Cancer.* Baltimore, Williams and Wilkins, 1983, p 492.
2. Pontes JE, Pescatori E, Connelly R, et al: Circulating cancer cells in renal cell carcinoma, EORTC Genitourinary Group monograph 9, *Renal Cell Carcinoma Metastasis.* New York, Alan R. Liss (in press).
3. Weiss L, Gilbert HA (eds): *Metastatic Inefficiency in Liver Metastasis.* Boston, GK Hall, 1982, p 126.
4. Beare JB, McDonald JR: Involvement of the renal capsule in surgically removed hypernephroma: A gross and histologic study. *J Urol* 1949; 61:857.
5. Chute R, Soutter L, Kerr WS, Jr: The value of thoracoabdominal incision in the removal of kidney tumors. *N Engl J Med* 1952; 241:951.
6. Foley FEB, Mulvaney WP, Richardson EJ, et al: Radical nephrectomy for neoplasm. *J Urol* 1952; 68:39.
7. Robson CJ, Churchill BM, Anderson W: The results of radical nephrectomy for renal cell carcinoma. *J Urol* 1969; 101:297.
8. Skinner DG, Colvin RB, Vermillion CD, et al: Diagnosis and management of renal cell carcinoma. A clinical and pathologic study of 309 cases. *Cancer* 1971; 28:1165.
9. Mintz ER, and Gaul EA: Kidney tumors: Some causes of poor end results. *NY J Med* 1939; 39:1405.
10. Humphreys GA, Foot NC: Survival of patients (235) following nephrectomy for renal cell and transitional cell tumors of the kidney. *J Urol* 1960; 83:815.
11. Priestley JT: Survival following the removal of malignant renal neoplasms. *JAMA* 1939; 113:902.

12. Kaufman JJ, Mims MM: Tumors of the kidney, in *Current Problems in Surgery.* Chicago, Year Book Medical Publishers, Inc, 1966, p 1.
13. Mostofi FK: Pathology and spread of renal carcinoma, in King JS, Jr (ed): *Renal Neoplasia.* Boston, Little, Brown & Co, 1967, p 41.
14. Middleton RG, Presto AJ III: Radical thoracoabdominal nephrectomy for renal cell carcinoma. *J Urol* 1973; 110:36.
15. Patel NP, Lavengood RW: Renal cell carcinoma: Natural history and results of treatment. *J Urol* 1978; 119:722.
16. de Kernion JB, Berry D: The diagnosis and treatment of renal cell carcinoma. *Cancer* 1980; 45:1947.
17. Parker AE: Studies on the main posterior lymph channels of the abdomen and their connections with the lymphatic of the genito-urinary system. *Am J Anat* 1935; 56:409.
18. Cockett ATK: Lymphatic network of the kidney. 1. Anatomic and physiologic considerations. *Urology* 1977; 9:125.
19. Cockett ATK, Roberts AP, Moore RS: Evidence for two intrarenal lymphatic networks. *Invest Urol* 1969; 7:266.
20. Lebrie SJ, Mayerson HS: Composition of renal lymph and its significance. *Proc Soc Exp Biol Med* 1959; 100:378.
21. Cockett ATK, Roberts AP, Moore RS: Renal lymphatic transport of fluid and solutes. *Invest Urol* 1969; 7:10.
22. Threefoot SA, Kent WT, Hatchett BF: Lymphaticovenous and lymphaticolymphatic communications demonstrated by plastic corrosion models of rats and postmortem lymphangiography in man. *J Lab Clin Med* 1963; 61:9.
23. Marshall FF, Powell KC: Lymphadenectomy for renal cell carcinoma: Anatomical and therapeutic considerations. *J Urol* 1982; 128:677.
24. Pizzocaro G: Lymphadenectomy in renal adenocarcinoma, *Tumors of the Kidney,* in deKernion JB, Pavone-Macaluso M (ed): Baltimore, Williams and Wilkins, 1986, p 75.
25. Beare JB, McDonald JR: Involvement of the renal capsule in surgically removed hypernephroma: A gross and histologic study. *J Urol* 1949; 61:857.
26. Chute R, Soutter L, Kerr WS, Jr: The value of thoracoabdominal incision in the removal of kidney tumors. *N Engl J Med* 1949; 241:951.
27. Foley FEB, Mulvaney WP, Richardson EJ, et al: Radical nephrectomy for neoplasm. *J Urol* 1952; 68:39.
28. Judd ES, Hand JR: Hypernephroma. *J Urol* 1929; 22:10.
29. Cabot H: The operative approach for malignant tumors of the kidney. *J Urol* 1925; 14:261.
30. Robson CJ, Churchill BM, Anderson W: The results of radical nephrectomy for renal cell carcinoma. *J Urol* 1969; 101:297.
31. Giuliani L, Martorana G, Giberti C, et al: Results of radical nephrectomy with extensive lymphadenectomy for renal cell carcinoma. *J Urol* 1983; 130:664.
32. Hulten L, Rosencrantz M, Seeman T, et al: Occurrence and localization of lymphnode metastases in renal carcinoma. *Scand J Urol Nephrol* 1969; 3:129.
33. Carl P, Klein U, Gebauer A, et al: The value of lymphography for TNM classification of renal carcinoma. *Eur Urol* 1977; 3:286.
34. Sigel A, Chlepas S, Schrott KM, et al: Die operation des Nierentumors. *Chirurg* 1981; 52:545.

35. Flocks RH, Kadesky MC: Malignant neoplasms of the kidney: An analysis of 353 patients followed five years or more. *J Urol* 1958; 79:196.
36. Rafla S: Renal cell carcinoma. Natural history and results of treatment. *Cancer* 1970; 25:26.
37. Middleton RG, Presto AJ III: Radical thoracoabdominal nephrectomy for renal cell carcinoma. *J Urol* 1973; 110:36.
38. Angervall L, Wahlquist L: Follow-up and prognosis of renal cell carcinoma in a series operated by perifascial nephrectomy combined with adrenalectomy and retroperitoneal lymphadenectomy. *Eur Urol* 1978; 4:13.
39. Waters WB, Richie JP: Aggressive surgical approach to renal cell carcinoma: Review of 130 cases. *J Urol* 1979; 122:306.
40. Peters PC, Brown GL: The role of lymphadenectomy in the management of renal cell carcinoma. *Urol Clin North Am* 1980; 7:705.
41. Siminovitch JP, Montie JE, Straffon RA: Lymphadenectomy in renal adenocarcinoma. *J Urol* 1982; 127:1090.
42. Skinner DG, Vermillion CD, Colvin RB: The surgical management of renal cell carcinoma. *J Urol* 1972; 107:705.
43. Waters CA, Lewis LG, Frontz WA: Radiation therapy of renal cortical neoplasms with special reference to preoperative irradiation. *South Med J* 1934; 27:290.
44. Bixler LC, Stenstom KW, Creevy CD: Malignant tumors of the kidney: Review of 117 cases. *Radiology* 1944; 42:329.
45. Richies EW, Griffiths IH, Thackray AC: New growth of the kidney and ureter (The BAUS series). *Br J Urol* 1951; 23:297.
46. Flocks RH, Kadesky MC: Malignant neoplasms of the kidney: An analysis of 353 patients followed five years or more. *J Urol* 1958; 79:196.
47. Richies E: The place of radiotherapy in the management of parenchymal carcinoma of the kidney. *J Urol* 1966; 95:313.
48. Del Regato JA, Kagan AR: Basic considerations in radiotherapy of renal carcinoma, in King JS, Jr (ed): *International Symposium of Renal Neoplasia*. Little, Brown & Co, 1967, p 547.
49. Peeling WB, Mantell BS, Shepheard BGF: Post-operative irradiation in the treatment of renal cell carcinoma. *Br J Urol* 1969; 41:23.
50. Finney R: The value of radiotherapy in the treatment of hypernephroma—A clinical trial. *Br J Urol* 1973; 45:258.
51. Cox CE, Lacy SS, Montgomery WG, et al: Renal adenocarcinoma: 28-year reviews with emphasis on rationale and feasibility of preoperative radiotherapy. *J Urol* 1970; 104:53.
52. Skinner DG, Vermillion CD, Colvin RB: The surgical management of renal cell carcinoma. *J Urol* 1972; 107:705.
53. Rafla S: Renal cell carcinoma. Natural history and results of treatment. *Cancer* 1970; 25:26.
54. Wiley AL, Jr, Wirtanen GW, Ansfield FJ, et al: Combined intra-arterial Actinomycin D and radiation therapy for surgically unresectable hypernephroma. *J Urol* 1975; 114:198.
55. Almgard LE, Fernstrom I, Haverling M, et al: Treatment of renal carcinoma by embolic occlusion of the renal circulation. *Br J Urol* 1973; 45:474.
56. Williams G: Angioinfarction in renal adenocarcinoma, in deKernion JB, Pavone-Macaluso M (eds): *Tumors of the Kidney*. Baltimore: Williams and Wilkins, 1986, p 75.

57. Lalli AF, Petersen N, Wallace S: Roentgen guided infarction of kidneys and lungs. *Radiology* 1969; 93:434.
58. Gianturco C, Anderson JH, Wallace S: Mechanical development for arterial occlusion. AJR 1975; 124:438.
59. Dotter CL, Goldman ML, Rosch J: Instant selective arterial occlusion with isobutyl 2 cyanoacrylate. *Radiology* 1975; 114:227.
60. Mee AD, Heap SW: Preoperative balloon occlusion of the renal artery for radical nephrectomy. *Br J Urol* 1978; 50:153.
61. Ellman BA, Green CE, Eigenbrodte E, et al: Renal infarction with absolute ethanol. *Invest Radiol* 1980; 15:318.
62. Turner RD, Rand RW, Bentson JR, et al: Ferromagnetic silicone necrosis of hypernephromas by selective vascular occlusion of the tumor—A new technique. *J Urol* 1975; 113:455.
63. Lang EK: Advanced renal cell carcinoma: Treatment by transcatheter embolization with inert material and radioactive particles. *Prog Clin Cancer* 1982; 8:299.
64. Swanson DA, Johnson DE, von Essenbach AC, et al: Angioinfarction plus nephrectomy for metastatic renal cell carcinoma. *J Urol* 1983; 130:449.
65. Pontes JE, Goldrosen M, Murphy GP: Immunological response to tumor ischemia in a murine renal cell carcinoma model. *Oncology* 1983; 40:63.
66. Gottesman JE, Crawford ED, Grossman HB, et al: Infarction-nephrectomy for metastatic renal carcinoma. A Southwest Oncology Group Study. *Urology* 1985; 25:248.
67. Feldman F, Casarella WJ, Dick HM, et al: Selective intraarterial embolization of bone tumors. A useful adjunct in the management of selected lesions. *AJR* 1975; 123:130.
68. Wallace S, Granmayeh M, deSantos LA, et al: Arterial occlusion of pelvic bone tumors. *Cancer* 1979; 43:322.
69. Varma J, Huben RP, Wajsman Z, et al: Therapeutic embolization of pelvic metastases of renal cell carcinoma. *J Urol* 1984; 131:647.
70. Kato T, Nemoto R, Mori H, et al: Arterial chemoembolization with Mitomycin C microcapsules in the treatment of primary or secondary carcinoma of the kidney, liver, bone and intrapelvic organs. *Cancer* 1981; 48:674.

4

Partial Nephrectomy

Andrew C. Novick, M.D.

Since the report of Robson et al[1] two decades ago, radical nephrectomy has been established as the optimal form of curative treatment for
localized RCC.[2] The classic description of this operation includes preliminary
ligation of the renal artery and vein, excision of the kidney outside Gerota's
fascia, removal of the ipsilateral adrenal gland, and the performance of a formal
regional lymphadenectomy from the aortic bifurcation to the crus of the diaphragm.[1] Notwithstanding the acknowledged clinical efficacy of radical nephrectomy, the importance of some of these surgical principles is now being
questioned.

Robey and Schellhammer[3] have shown that routine ipsilateral adrenalectomy is not always necessary, particularly with lower pole RCCs. Because nodal
metastasis is associated with poor extended survival,[4] removal of regional lymph
nodes has prognostic value. The therapeutic benefit of lymphadenectomy as yet
is unproved, and there remains no effective adjuvant treatment for patients in
whom positive nodes are found. Although preliminary ligation of the major
renal vessels is an accepted and practiced tenet, this measure does not necessarily
assure complete control of the kidney's blood supply, particularly with large
tumors that often have abundant collateral vasculature. The finding of perinephric fat invasion in approximately 25% of patients with RCC provides a sound
basis for performing perifascial nephrectomy to minimize the potential for local
spillage of tumor cells. Although the risk of local tumor recurrence after radical
nephrectomy appears to be small, the exact incidence is not known presently.

These arguments surrounding various aspects of radical nephrectomy have
been rendered even more relevant and controversial by recent data concerning
patient outcome after partial nephrectomy for RCC. This approach was initially
limited to patients with localized carcinoma present bilaterally or in a solitary
kidney, in whom radical nephrectomy would necessitate immediate renal replacement therapy. Several reports[5-11] of excellent long-term cancer-free survival
in such cases have encouraged expansion of the indications for partial neph-

rectomy in RCC. Other developments that have impacted on this issue include improved surgical techniques that now allow large tumors to be completely excised with preservation of uninvolved parenchyma[12] and the increasing discovery of "incidental" RCCs on noninvasive imaging studies (CT, magnetic resonance imaging, ultrasonography) obtained for other conditions[13]; the latter are generally small, peripheral, low stage lesions and may be more amenable to local excision.

NEPHROLOGIC CONSIDERATIONS

An intriguing nephrologic issue has been raised by recent data suggesting that loss of a critical mass of renal tissue may result in accelerated progressive loss of function of the remaining tissue because of the development of focal and segmental glomerular sclerosis. This concern arose initially because of studies[14–16] in rats in which renal ablation led to albuminuria, hypertension, and progressive renal dysfunction presumably as a result of hyperfiltration in remaining tissue. The theoretic extrapolation of these findings with animals to the human situation has generated both considerable controversy and the search for a clinical correlate. The observation of an increased incidence of focal glomerular sclerosis in the contralateral kidney of patients with unilateral renal agenesis may represent one such example.[17] Several studies have evaluated long-term renal function in kidney donors after nephrectomy as another human model. Some of these studies,[18, 19] although not all,[20, 21] have found a greater frequency of hypertension and mild proteinuria in such donors. This information raises the possibility that patients undergoing a unilateral nephrectomy may be at risk for developing slowly progressive loss of function in the remaining kidney. Validation of this concept would provide further impetus to consider nephron-sparing surgery in RCC, perhaps even in patients with a completely normal opposite kidney. It is appropriate to emphasize that this issue is presently unresolved and remains the focus of further clinical studies.

As indicated previously, increasingly sophisticated surgical techniques now allow large localized RCCs to be completely excised while preserving the blood supply and urinary drainage for a relatively small portion of tumor-free parenchyma. This raises the nephrologic consideration concerning the minimal amount of viable parenchyma necessary to sustain adequate renal function without dialysis in patients with carcinoma involving a solitary kidney. It is well known that after loss of renal mass the remaining nephrons undergo functional and structural hypertrophy. The extent of this compensatory increase in renal mass, renal blood flow, and single nephron glomerular filtration rate is directly proportional to the amount of renal tissue removed.[22, 23] Age is no barrier to the development of compensatory hypertrophy, but this process is more pronounced in younger patients.

We have found that satisfactory overall renal function can ultimately be achieved with as little as 15% to 20% of one kidney. In such cases early post-

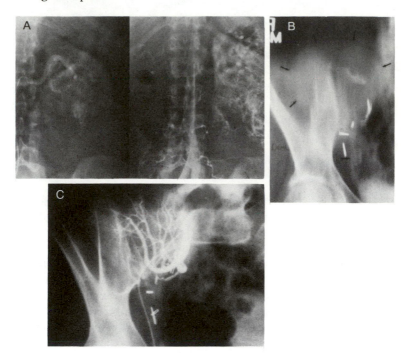

FIG 4–1.
A, left renal arteriogram shows large vascular carcinoma involving lower three fourths of solitary left kidney. The tumor was completely excised extracorporeally, and 15% to 20% of the kidney (upper pole) was salvaged. After autotransplantation, renal function was initially poor but improved gradually. **B,** 1 year after operation IV pyelogram shows good function of the hypertrophic renal remnant. The serum creatinine level at this time is 2.3 mg/dL. **C,** arteriogram demonstrates excellent blood supply to the renal autograft. (From Novick AC: *Urol Clin North Am* 1987; 14:419. Used by permission.)

operative function of the renal remnant is often suboptimal, occasionally requiring temporary dialysis. Gradually, with resolution of postischemic acute tubular nephrosis and the initiation of hypertrophy, renal function begins to improve. Although the greatest degree of hypertrophy and recovery of renal function occurs within the first 3 months after surgery, this process often continues for up to 24 months with further gradual lowering of the serum creatinine level during this period (Fig 4–1).

PATIENT SELECTION

Bilateral Renal Cell Carcinoma

The incidence of bilateral RCC is approximately 2% with an equal number of synchronous and asynchronous presentations. Partial nephrectomy is well

TABLE 4–1.
Survival After Partial Versus Radical Nephrectomy in
Unilateral RCC

SERIES (YR)	TYPE OF NEPHRECTOMY	5-YR SURVIVAL (%)
Robson (1969)	Radical	66*
Skinner (1971)	Radical	68*
Marberger (1981)	Partial	78
Novick (1988)	Partial	77
*Stage I tumors only.		

established as the treatment of choice for patients in this category with localized malignancy that is amenable to complete surgical excision.

Patients with localized synchronous bilateral RCC have an interesting dilemma in terms of the approach to partial nephrectomy. Most of these patients are in the fifth or sixth decade, are otherwise healthy, and have a life expectancy of 10 to 20 years if they remain free of malignancy. In general, operative therapy should be oriented toward preserving as much tumor-free renal parenchyma as possible to guard against either a renal-threatening surgical complication or the development later in life of a disorder that impairs renal function. Therefore it is appropriate to consider performing bilateral partial nephrectomies if these are technically feasible. In general, it is more prudent to stage these operations unless one or both kidneys are involved with a single small tumor. When one of the involved kidneys is extensively replaced by tumor, a radical nephrectomy on that side and a contralateral partial nephrectomy are indicated. In this situation, it is also more prudent to stage these operations by first performing the partial nephrectomy and when a good surgical result is assured, removing the contralateral kidney. This sequence obviates the need for temporary dialysis if reversible postischemic renal failure occurs after the partial nephrectomy.

Unilateral Renal Cell Carcinoma

Partial nephrectomy is the treatment of choice for patients with localized unilateral RCC involving a solitary kidney. Because unilateral renal agenesis or hypoplasia is rare, occurring in only one of 600 live births, most patients in this category will either have undergone removal of the opposite kidney or that kidney will have been rendered nonfunctioning as a result of a benign disease process. Excellent long-term cancer-free survival has been reported after partial nephrectomy in such patients with unilateral RCC, and these results are comparable to those reported after radical nephrectomy for low stage RCC (Table 4–1). On the basis of these data, the indications for nephron-sparing surgery have been extended to include patients with localized RCC and a functioning opposite kidney when that kidney is involved with a disorder (e.g., calculi, diabetes, nephrosclerosis, pyelonephritis, arterial disease, hydronephrosis) that might cause progressive renal functional impairment in the future.

There is currently controversy concerning the role of partial nephrectomy in patients with unilateral RCC and a normal opposite kidney with no intercurrent condition that might subsequently impair the function of that kidney. There are now reports[24] of nephron-sparing surgery being performed in such patients for small peripheral RCCs, particularly those that are incidentally discovered. Presently the indications for partial nephrectomy in patients with a completely normal opposite kidney are not established, and radical nephrectomy must still be considered the treatment of choice in this setting.

Renal Cell Carcinoma in von Hippel-Lindau Disease

von Hippel-Lindau disease is one of the phakomatoses that constitutes retinal hemangiomas, central nervous system hemangioblastomas, and cystic disease of multiple organs. RCC is known to occur in approximately 45% of patients with von Hippel-Lindau disease.[25] RCC in von Hippel-Lindau disease differs from its sporadic counterpart in several important aspects. It usually is diagnosed earlier in life (third to fifth decades), and there is only a slight male predominance instead of the normal 3:1 male to female ratio. Perhaps most important, there is a tendency toward multicentricity with RCC in von Hippel-Lindau disease, which most often is manifested by multiple bilateral solid and/or cystic tumors. These tumors are capable of progression with metastasis, and in a large series by Horton et al,[26] 32% of the patients with von Hippel-Lindau disease died of RCC.

Nephron-sparing surgery is indicated for patients with localized bilateral RCC and von Hippel-Lindau disease.[25, 27, 28] Surgical treatment in these patients must include the recognition that all renal cysts in von Hippel-Lindau disease are potentially malignant.[29] A consistent and characteristic histologic feature in von Hippel-Lindau disease is the presence of clear cells lining cysts with or without frank carcinoma within the renal cyst walls; these cysts are incipient RCCs (Fig 4–2). For this reason, adequate treatment can only be assured by excising all cystic and solid renal lesions identified on preoperative radiographic studies and/or at surgery. In view of the multicentric nature of RCC in von Hippel-Lindau disease, one may not be entirely certain of having removed microscopic or clinically undetectable small intraparenchymal lesions. This concern underscores the importance of close postoperative surveillance with CT scanning to allow early diagnosis and prompt treatment of newly identified lesions.

We[25] recently reported a group of 10 patients with von Hippel-Lindau disease who underwent surgical treatment for nonmetastatic bilateral RCC. Nephron-sparing surgery was performed in nine patients, whereas one patient with extensive tumor replacement of both kidneys underwent bilateral nephrectomy with subsequent hemodialysis and renal allotransplantation. Of the nine patients who underwent partial nephrectomy, eight were alive with good renal function and no evidence of malignancy.

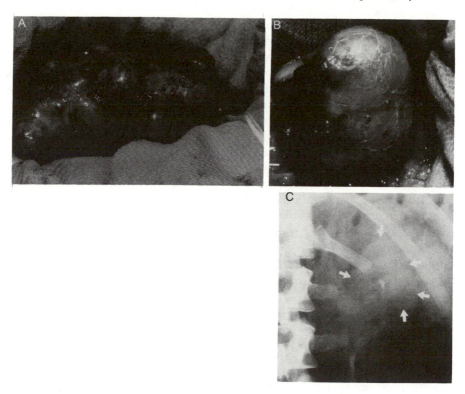

FIG 4–2.
A, operative photograph of kidney involved with multiple cystic and solid lesions in patient with von Hippel-Lindau disease. **B,** operative photograph of the remaining upper third of the kidney after in situ excision of all tumors, after circulation has been restored. **C,** postoperative IV urogram shows good function of the remaining portion of the left kidney. (**A** from Spencer WF, Novick AC, Montie JE, et al: *J Urol* 1988; 139:507. **B** and **C** from Novick AC: *Urol Clin North Am* 1987; 14:419. Used by permission.)

SURGICAL TECHNIQUES

Patients undergoing partial nephrectomy for RCC should be studied pre-operatively with standard catheter renal arteriography to delineate the main renal artery and its branches. Knowledge of the number and location of these vessels helps greatly in removing the tumor with minimal blood loss and injury to adjacent parenchyma. In patients with a large or centrally located RCC, renal venography is a useful study even when there are no clinical or radiographic findings to suggest IVC involvement. Renal venography in such cases is indicated to determine whether an intrarenal venous tumor thrombus is present. The latter implies a more advanced tumor stage with a diminished prognosis for the patient and also renders the task of performing partial nephrectomy more technically complicated (Fig 4–3).

In patients undergoing partial nephrectomy for RCC, every attempt should be made to minimize intraoperative ischemic renal damage. Vigorous intravenous fluid hydration should be initiated before surgery to ensure optimal renal perfusion in the operating room. Important general intraoperative measures include prevention of hypotension, administration of mannitol, and avoidance of traction or excessive manipulation of the renal artery. When the renal circulation is temporarily interrupted, local hypothermia offers the most effective technique for protection against ischemic renal injury. Clamping of the renal artery alone is also less ischemia-rendering than clamping the entire renal pedicle, since maintaining renal venous patency allows retrograde perfusion and oxygenation of the kidney.

The specific techniques for performing partial nephrectomy in RCC are described in detail elsewhere.[12] All these techniques require adherence to basic principles of early vascular control, avoidance of ischemic renal damage, complete tumor excision with free margins, precise closure of the collecting system, careful hemostasis, and closure or coverage of the renal defect with adjacent fat, fascia, peritoneum, or oxidized cellulose.

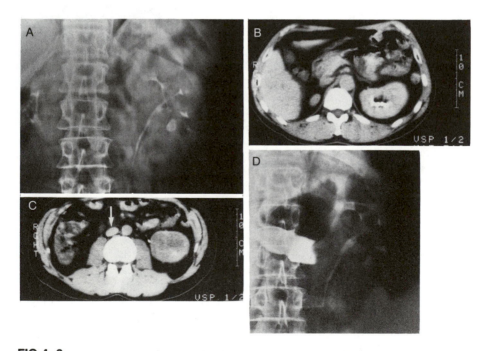

FIG 4–3.
A, IV pyelogram shows hypoplastic right kidney and large mass involving the lower half of the left kidney. **B,** CT scan section through the upper part of the left kidney shows no renal carcinoma at this level. **C,** CT scan section through the middle of the left kidney shows extensive replacement with carcinoma. The vena cava is well demonstrated (*arrow*) and appears normal. **D,** left renal venography shows occlusion of the left main renal vein, which was due to a tumor thrombus.

In most cases it is possible to perform partial nephrectomy for RCC in situ with an operative approach that optimizes exposure of the kidney and by combining meticulous surgical technique with an understanding of the renal vascular anatomy in relation to the tumor. We employ an extraperitoneal flank incision through the bed of rib 11 or 12 for all these operations. This incision allows the surgeon to operate on the mobilized kidney almost at skin level and provides excellent exposure of the peripheral renal vessels. With an anterior transperitoneal incision, the kidney is invariably located in the depth of the wound, and the surgical exposure is less satisfactory.

When performing partial nephrectomy for RCC in situ, the kidney is mobilized inside Gerota's fascia; however, the perirenal fat around the tumor is left undisturbed. When the tumor is confined to the upper or lower pole of the kidney, partial nephrectomy can be done by ligating the segmental apical or basilar arterial branch and excising the involved renal segment at the observed line of demarcation, while allowing unimpaired perfusion to the rest of the kidney from the main renal artery. Excision of nonpolar tumors is most effectively performed after temporary renal arterial occlusion. The most commonly employed techniques in such cases involve a wedge or transverse renal resection with appropriate reconstruction of the remaining portion of the kidney.

Enucleation

There is controversy concerning the technique of simple enucleation in patients undergoing nephron-sparing surgery for RCC. In 1950, Vermooten[30] reported that some RCCs are completely enveloped by a distinct pseudocapsule of fibrous tissue that renders them amenable to excision by surgical enucleation. Subsequent reports, however, have offered conflicting data regarding the safety and efficacy of this technique. Favorable results have been reported by Graham and Glenn,[31] Carini et al,[32] and Jaeger et al[33] and in a combined study from the Mayo and Cleveland Clinics.[34] Other histopathologic and clinical studies[35-37] have highlighted the risk of leaving residual malignancy in the kidney operated on when enucleation is performed; in one series, three cases of postoperative tumor recurrence were directly ascribed to the use of this technique.[7]

It has become clear that the basis for these discrepant experiences is the difficulty in assuring complete tumor encapsulation before undertaking enucleation. Because excision of a margin of normal renal cortex around a carcinoma does not generally increase the technical difficulty of surgery, this is now the recommended approach for most patients. Surgical enucleation is currently indicated only in patients with von Hippel-Lindau disease who have multiple diffuse carcinomas or patients with an encapsulated hilar tumor (in a solitary kidney) that directly overlies the major renal vessels with no interposed margin of uninvolved parenchyma.

Extracorporeal Tumor Excision

Extracorporeal partial nephrectomy is an important surgical advance that has enabled removal of complex renal tumors previously considered inoperable.[12] The advantages of an extracorporeal approach in this setting include optimal exposure, a bloodless surgical field, the ability to perform a more precise operation with maximal conservation of renal parenchyma, and greater protection of the kidney from prolonged ischemia.

In a recent report from our center,[38] ex vivo surgery was performed in 14 of 100 patients undergoing partial nephrectomy for RCC from 1956 to 1987. We observed that ex vivo tumor excision has been necessary less often in recent years with only two of 58 patients (3.4%) managed in this fashion since 1983. Although there are certainly some large, hypervascular, centrally located RCCs that can only be excised with an ex vivo approach, such cases appear to be quite uncommon. In our study the incidence of temporary ($p = 0.0005$) and permanent ($p = 0.05$) renal failure was significantly greater after ex vivo excision than with in situ excision. Therefore an ex vivo approach should only be employed when necessary and when backup dialysis support is available. The efficacy of extracorporeal partial nephrectomy in such cases is attested to by the fact that despite its use in more complex and locally extensive RCCs, the postoperative survival and local tumor recurrence rates are equivalent to those obtained in patients managed in situ.[38]

RESULTS OF PARTIAL NEPHRECTOMY FOR RENAL CELL CARCINOMA

Patient Survival

There are no concurrent data comparing survival after radical versus partial nephrectomy for RCCs of comparable pathologic stage and size. Nevertheless, there are now several reports of excellent long-term cancer-free survival after partial nephrectomy for RCC, and these results are equivalent to those reported after radical nephrectomy for low stage RCC. We[38] recently reviewed our experience with partial nephrectomy as curative therapy for RCC in 100 consecutive patients; this series included 56 patients with bilateral RCC (28 synchronous, 28 asynchronous) and 44 patients with unilateral RCC. The 5-year survival rate for patients in the entire series was 67% including death from any cause and 84% including only deaths from RCC. The corresponding 5-year survival rates for patients in stage 1 RCC (n = 75) were 73% and 90%, respectively. These data support the emerging view that partial nephrectomy does not significantly compromise the long-term survival of patients with low stage RCC.

Several earlier reports had suggested diminished survival after partial nephrectomy in patients with bilateral asynchronous RCC compared with those with unilateral or bilateral synchronous RCC.[9-11] In our abovementioned recent review, the 5-year survival rates for patients with unilateral RCC were significantly better than those for bilateral synchronous or asynchronous RCC ($p < 0.5$); survival in the latter two subgroups with bilateral RCC was not significantly different. Consonant with these observed differences in survival, a significantly diminished incidence of postoperative tumor recurrence was observed in patients with unilateral RCC compared with those with bilateral synchronous or asynchronous RCC ($p < 0.0005$). Although the approach to therapy remains the same for patients with localized unilateral or bilateral RCC who require nephron-sparing surgery, these observations are nonetheless interesting. They suggest that in some patients with bilateral RCC the second renal tumor may represent the initial manifestation of metastatic disease.

Postoperative Renal Function

In our review of partial nephrectomy for RCC in 100 patients, the preoperative serum creatinine levels ranged from 0.9 to 3.7 mg dL (mean 1.44 mg/dL), and postoperative renal function was carefully evaluated. Ninety-three patients (93%) experienced immediate function of the kidney operated on, whereas seven patients (7%) required dialysis postoperatively because of initial nonfunction of the repaired kidney. Four of these patients ultimately achieved satisfactory renal function after resolution of postischemic renal failure; in the remaining three patients there was no recovery of function, and long-term dialysis was maintained. Therefore in the overall series preservation of renal function was achieved in 97 patients (97%) after partial nephrectomy for RCC. The postoperative serum creatinine levels in these patients ranged from 0.9 to 4.6 mg/dL (mean 1.76 mg/dL). Currently, partial nephrectomy for RCC can be performed with a high degree of success in achieving the goal of preserving functioning tumor-free renal parenchyma.

Local Tumor Recurrence

Patients who undergo partial nephrectomy for RCC must be followed closely for local tumor recurrence in the treated kidney, which has been reported in 9% to 13% of patients.[6, 9-11] This represents the major disadvantage of partial nephrectomy compared with radical nephrectomy. The risk of local recurrence after radical nephrectomy has not been determined but is presumably much less since (1) the diseased kidney has been removed and is no longer at risk for developing recurrent cancer; and (2) Gerota's fascia is kept intact during the operation, which theoretically reduces the risk of tumor spillage.

CT scanning is presently the most accurate diagnostic method for detecting locally recurrent RCC after partial nephrectomy, and this should be done at least every 6 months after operation to ensure an early diagnosis. Patients who develop a local recurrence with no signs of metastasis may be considered for secondary surgical treatment, which in our experience is possible in approximately 50% of cases.[39] In some patients, another partial nephrectomy can be done to achieve complete tumor excision with preservation of renal function and the opportunity for extended survival. If this is not technically possible, total nephrectomy with initiation of long-term dialysis then offers the only possibility for curative treatment. Patients who subsequently remain tumor-free on dialysis for a minimal period of 15 months may undergo renal allotransplantation to restore renal function.[40] In some cases local tumor recurrence after partial nephrectomy occurs concomitantly with the development of metastatic disease, and the prognosis for these patients is poor.

SUMMARY

In recent years partial nephrectomy has been established as an effective approach for patients with localized RCC in whom preservation of functioning renal parenchyma is a relevant clinical consideration. The technical success rate is high, and long-term cancer-free patient survival is comparable to that obtained after radical nephrectomy, particularly for low stage tumors. The major disadvantage of partial nephrectomy is the approximately 10% risk of postoperative local tumor recurrence. The risk of local recurrence after radical nephrectomy has not been determined but is presumably less. The indications for partial nephrectomy in patients with unilateral RCC and a completely normal opposite kidney are not established, and radical nephrectomy must still be considered the treatment of choice in this setting. The role of partial nephrectomy may be modified further in the future as effective systemic therapy becomes available for patients with RCC.

REFERENCES

1. Robson CJ, Churchill BM, Andrew W: The results of radical nephrectomy for renal cell carcinoma. *J Urol* 1969; 101:297.
2. Skinner DG, Colvin RB, Vermillion CD, et al: Diagnosis and management of renal cell carcinoma: A clinical and pathological study of 309 cases. *Cancer* 1971; 28:1165.
3. Robey EL, Schellhammer PF: The adrenal gland and renal cell carcinoma. Is ipsilateral adrenalectomy a necessary component of radical nephrectomy. *J Urol* 1986; 135:453.
4. Siminovitch JP, Montie JE, Straffon RA: Lymphadenectomy in renal adenocarcinoma. *J Urol* 1982; 127:1090.
5. Schiff M, Bagley DH, Lytton B: Treatment of solitary and bilateral renal carcinomas. *J Urol* 1979; 121:581.
6. Topley M, Novick AC, Montie JE: Long-term results following partial nephrectomy for localized renal adenocarcinoma. *J Urol* 1984; 131:1050.
7. Smith RB, de Kernion JB, Ehrlich RM, et al: Bilateral renal cell carcinoma and renal cell carcinoma in the solitary kidney. *J Urol* 1984; 132:450.
8. Zincke H, Engen DE, Henning KM, et al: Treatment of renal cell carcinoma by in situ partial nephrectomy and extracorporeal operation with autotransplantation. *Mayo Clin Proc* 1985; 60:651.

9. Zincke H, Swanson SK: Bilateral renal cell carcinoma: Influence of synchronous and asynchronous occurrence on patient survival. *J Urol* 1982; 128:913.
10. Jacobs SC, Berg SI, Lawson RK: Synchronous bilateral renal cell carcinoma: Total surgical excision. *Cancer* 1980; 46:2341.
11. Marberger M, Pugh RCB, Auvert J, et al: Conservative surgery of renal carcinoma: The EIRSS Experience. *Br J Urol* 1981; 53:528.
12. Novick AC: Partial nephrectomy for renal cell carcinoma. *Urol Clin North Am* 1987; 14:419.
13. Konnak JW, Grossman HB: Renal cell carcinoma as an incidental finding. *J Urol* 1985; 134:1094.
14. Shimamura T, Morrison AB: A progressive glomerulosclerosis occurring in partial five-sixths nephrectomized rats. *Am J Pathol* 1975; 79:95.
15. Hostetter TH, Olson JL, Rennke HG, et al: Hyperfiltration in remnant nephrons: A potentially adverse response to renal ablation. *Am J Physiol* 1981; 241:F85.
16. Brenner BM, Meyer TW, Hostetter TH: Dietary protein intake and the progressive natures of kidney disease: The role of hemodynamically mediated glomerular injury in the pathogenesis of progressive glomerular sclerosis in aging, renal ablation, and intrinsic renal disease. *N Engl J Med* 1982; 307:652.
17. Kiprov DD, Colvin RB, McCluskey RT: Focal and sequential glomerulosclerosis and proteinuria associated with unilateral renal agenesis. *Lab Invest* 1982; 46:275.
18. Goldszer RC, Hakim RM, Brenner BM: Long-term follow-up of renal function in kidney transplant donors. *Kidney Int* 1983; 23:124.
19. Miller IJ, Suthanthiran M, Riggio RR, et al: Impact of renal donation: Long-term clinical and biochemical follow-up of living donors in a single center. *Am J Med* 1985; 79:201.
20. Vincenti F, Amend WJC, Kaysen G, et al: Long-term renal function in kidney donors: Sustained compensatory hyperfiltration with no adverse effects. *Transplantation* 1983; 36:626.
21. Anderson CF, Velosa JA, Frohnert PP, et al: The risks of unilateral nephrectomy: Status of kidney donors 10 to 20 years postoperatively. *Mayo Clin Proc* 1985; 60:367.
22. Kaufman JM, DiMeola HJ, Siegel NJ, et al: Compensatory adaptation of structure and function following progressive renal ablation. *Kidney Int* 1974; 6:10.
23. Hayslett JP: Effect of age on compensatory renal growth. *Kidney Int* 1983; 23:599.
24. Bazeed MA, Scharfe T, Becht E, et al: Conservative surgery of renal cell carcinoma. *Eur Urol* 1986; 12:238.
25. Spencer WF, Novick AC, Montie JE, et al: Surgical treatment of localized renal cell carcinoma in von Hippel-Lindau disease. *J Urol* 1988; 139:507.
26. Horton WA, Wong V, Eldridge R: von Hippel-Lindau disease: Clinical and pathological manifestations in nine families with 50 affected members. *Arch Intern Med* 1976; 136:769.
27. Pearson JC, Weiss J, Tanagho EA: A plea for conservation of kidneys in renal adenocarcinoma associated with von Hippel-Lindau disease. *J Urol* 1980; 124:910.
28. Loughlin KR, Gittes RF: Urological management of patients with von Hippel-Lindau disease. *J Urol* 1986; 136:789.
29. Christenson PJ, Craig JP, Bibbo MC, et al: Cysts containing renal cell carcinoma in von Hippel-Lindau disease. *J Urol* 1982; 128:798.
30. Vermooten V: Indications for conservative surgery in certain renal tumors: A study based on the growth pattern of clear cell carcinoma. *J Urol* 1950; 64:200.

31. Graham SD, Glenn JF: Enucleative surgery for renal malignancy. *J Urol* 1979; 122:546.
32. Carini M, Selli C, Muraro GB, et al: Conservative surgery for renal cell carcinoma. *Eur Urol* 1981; 7:19.
33. Jaeger N, Weissbach L, Vahlensieck W: Value of enucleation of tumor in solitary kidneys. *Eur Urol* 1985; 11:369.
34. Novick AC, Zincke H, Neves RJ, et al: Surgical enucleation for renal cell carcinoma. *J Urol* 1986; 135:235.
35. Marshall FF, Taxy JB, Fishman EK, et al: The feasibility of surgical enucleation for renal cell carcinoma. *J Urol* 1986; 135:231.
36. Rosenthal CL, Kraft R, Zingg EJ: Organ-preserving surgery in renal cell carcinoma: tumor enucleation versus partial kidney resection. *Eur Urol* 1984; 10:222.
37. Blackley SK, Ladaga L, Woolfitt RA, et al: Ex situ study of the effectiveness of enucleation in patients with renal cell carcinoma. *J Urol* 1988; 140:6.
38. Novick AC, Streem SB, Montie JE, et al: Conservative surgery for renal cell carcinoma: A single-center experience with 100 patients. *J Urol.* 1989; 141:835.
39. Novick AC, Straffon RA: Management of locally recurrent renal cell carcinoma following partial nephrectomy. *J Urol* 1987; 138:603.
40. Penn I: Transplantation in patients with primary renal malignancies. *Transplantation* 1977; 24:424.

5

Inferior Vena Cava Tumor Thrombectomy

James E. Montie, M.D.

Renal tumors are unique in oncology in their propensity to propagate in large veins without true invasion of the vein. RCC is by far the most common carcinoma demonstrating this phenomenon; however, a tumor thrombus may also be seen with other types of renal parenchyma tumors. Therefore it is not clear if this growth pattern is a result of intrarenal hemodynamics or a peculiarity of the growth characteristics of RCC. Renal vein and IVC tumor thrombus extensions have been seen with Wilms' tumors, adrenocortical cancers involving the kidney, and other renal sarcomas. The fact that carcinomas in the renal parenchyma can invade blood vessels, form a tumor thrombus in the renal vein, grow into the lumen of the IVC, and still not demonstrate metastases is a fascinating observation in cancer biology, one that has not been explored. In most other epithelial carcinomas, even microscopic vascular invasion is associated with a strong prediction of later or concurrent distant metastases. With RCC extensions into the IVC, the number of tumor cells that are continually shed into the circulation must be tremendous. The absence of pulmonary metastases in any of these patients is noteworthy and was even commented on 45 years ago by McDonald and Priestly.[1] Are the tumor cells that are shed nonviable, unable to establish a metastasis, or is the lung an unfavorable environment? Because the lungs are one of the most common sites of metastases for RCC, more specific research is needed on the biology of RCC relative to invasion and implantation of metastases and on pulmonary defense mechanisms in this system.

BACKGROUND

The ability of RCC to propagate in the lumen of the renal vein and IVC has been recognized for many years. Resection of an IVC thrombus at the time of radical nephrectomy for RCC was reported as early as 1913 by Berg.[2] Until the advent of arteriography and phlebography in the 1940s and 1950s, the IVC involvement was discovered only at the time of surgery. The surgeon was generally unprepared or not trained to use necessary vascular techniques to safely remove the thrombus; the procedure was either abandoned or the kidney removed with the thrombus left indwelling. As early as 1924, a fatal intraoperative tumor embolus was described.[3] Although involvement of the renal vein was recognized from surgical pathology and autopsy studies, McDonald and Priestly[1] described in 1943 the prognostic significance of renal vein and IVC invasion, likening it to the adverse impact on survival imposed by lymph node metastases. These observations contributed to the inclusion of right ventricular involvement in stage III along with regional lymph nodes in the staging system of Robson et al,[4] which still is widely used today. With the development of IVC phlebography, the presence of the thrombus in the IVC could be identified preoperatively, allowing the surgeon the luxury of planning for the vascular aspects of the operation. However, the poor prognosis believed to be associated with IVC involvement and a significant increase in the complexity of the procedure led most urologists to consider aggressive surgical treatment ill-advised.

Evidence presented in the early 1970s suggested that at least some segment of patients with an IVC tumor thrombus could have an extended disease-free survival if the kidney and all the thrombi were removed.[5] The absence of any other remotely effective treatment and increasing sophistication of the surgical technique gradually prompted a more aggressive surgical approach to be adopted in larger centers. The relatively low frequency of IVC involvement made it difficult for large series to be accumulated, and it was not until the late 1970s and 1980s that more than anecdotal data were available. As recently as 1985, the isolated case report of a successful removal of tumor thrombus in the atrium was considered worthy of publication.[6] A cumulative series of 69 patients at the Cleveland Clinic Foundation between 1956 and 1987 with an IVC tumor thrombus resected is the largest single institution experience available.[7,8] Many of the observations reported herein are based on a recent review from the Cleveland Clinic Foundation.[8]

INCIDENCE

There are approximately 20,000 new cases of RCC yearly in the United States. Gross renal vein invasion occurs in approximately 30%, involvement of the IVC in approximately 5%, and extension to the diaphragm or atrium in 0.05% to 1%. Thus there are approximately 1,000 cases per year of RCC with IVC extension. Many of these (30% to 40%) will have metastases at the time of diagnosis commonly associated with a poor performance status and thus will not even be considered for surgery. These figures are based on data from major medical centers and not from population-based registries and thus may not be entirely reflective of the general population.

PREOPERATIVE EVALUATION

To properly plan an operation on an RCC tumor thrombus, the presence and extent of the thrombus must be known preoperatively. As imaging technology has advanced in recent years, the options available to study the renal vein and the IVC have increased (see Chapter 2).

One cannot rely on symptoms to select patients with IVC involvement. Published series[9, 10] indicated that only 7% to 25% of patients with IVC thrombus had any symptoms such as peripheral edema, deep venous thrombosis, renal insufficiency, pulmonary embolus, or ascites. A recent review of 48 patients at Cleveland Clinic Foundation identified 16% with symptoms suggesting IVC involvement.

Some authors have recommended inferior venacavography in all patients with RCC to be sure a tumor thrombus was not present. This is unnecessary, but it is appropriate to ensure patency of the renal vein by *some* technique before the operation.[11] Tumor thrombus in the renal vein alone does not require modification of the surgical technique; however, if we are sure there is not a thrombus in the renal vein, we can essentially eliminate the possibility of an IVC thrombus (a rare case has been reported with IVC thrombus propagating through only one of several renal veins).

An intravenous pyelogram (IVP) alone is not enough to rule out an IVC thrombus. The absence of these findings does not guarantee that a thrombus is not present, but some clues on a urogram can identify patients at high risk for IVC involvement (see Fig 2–15). Right-sided tumors, large central carcinomas, and nonvisualization of the kidney on contrast studies are increasingly associated with renal vein and IVC involvement. Ultrasonography and abdominal CT have been reported to be effective in identifying the presence of a renal vein or IVC thrombus. Magnetic resonance imaging is extremely valuable but unlikely to be used widely now as an initial study because of cost and logistic considerations. A thrombus in the renal vein and IVC frequently receives its blood supply from the renal artery, thus a characteristic "blush" can be seen on the late arterial phase of a renal arteriogram (see Figure 2–34). Conversely, the brisk arteriovenous shunting in an RCC can often be seen on an angiogram, and the renal vein can be identified as patent on an early venous phase of this study (see Fig 2–31). It is the surgeon's responsibility to be confident by some imaging studies that IVC is not involved before proceeding with the operation.

If a thrombus is identified in the IVC, the next step is to precisely define the extent of the thrombus. A categorization of four levels advocated by the Mayo Clinic has been adopted and is valuable because the defined levels cor-

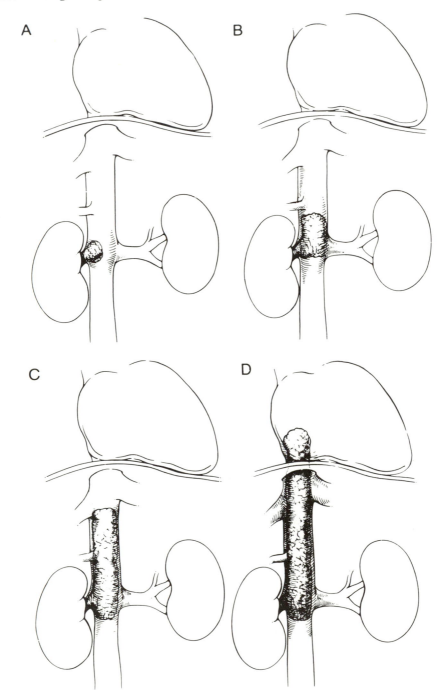

FIG 5–1.
The four levels of IVC involvement corresponding to definitions in Table 5–1. **A,** level I. **B,** level II. **C,** level III. **D,** level IV. (From Novick AC, Montie JE: Surgery for renal cell carcinoma involving the inferior vena cava, in Novick AC, Streem SS, Pontes JE [eds]: *Stewart's Operative Urology.* Baltimore, Williams and Wilkins Co, 1989. Used by permission.)

TABLE 5–1.
Level of IVC Involvement

LEVEL OF THROMBUS	OPERATIVE TECHNIQUE
I. Renal: <2 cm from renal ostia	Satinsky clamp on IVC
II. Infrahepatic: >2 cm from renal ostia but below main hepatic veins	Control of IVC above thrombus but below hepatic veins, contralateral renal vein, IVC below tumor thrombus, lumbar veins
III. Intrahepatic: intrahepatic IVC, below diaphragm	Control of IVC at diaphragm, porta hepatis, superior mesenteric artery, inferior mesenteric artery, renal vein, IVC below tumor thrombus, lumbar veins, or cardiac bypass with or without circulatory arrest
IV. Supradiaphragmatic or atrial	Cardiac bypass with or without circulatory arrest

respond with modifications needed in the surgical technique (Fig 5–1, Table 5–1).[9] Other classifications have used three levels, essentially by combining the renal and infrahepatic levels.[12]

An inferior venacavogram has been the mainstay of delineating the extent of the thrombus. A small thrombus will appear as a filling defect in the opacified lumen of the IVC (see Figure 2–30). Occasionally a false-positive study can be seen as a result of flow artifact created by unopacified blood streaming from the ipsilateral renal vein, distortion caused by a retrocaval or precaval lymph node, or distortion from a medial extension of the tumor in the kidney (see Figure 2–32).

Usually additional imaging studies can help clarify the situation. A long thin "tail" of a thrombus can sometimes be so small that the uppermost extent is underestimated (Fig 5–2). It is extremely important to be certain of the caudal extent of the thrombus. When a thrombus causes significant hemodynamic obstruction in the IVC, collateral circulation will begin to be evident in existing but normally underdeveloped networks with the azygous system (Figs 5–3 and 5–4). The insidious growth pattern of the tumor thrombus usually allows this collateral circulation to be extensive; clinical evidence of venous insufficiency below the thrombus is uncommon (see Fig 2–3). When edema or deep venous thrombosis of the lower extremity is seen, it is generally associated with nontumorous thrombus propagation into the iliac or femoral veins (see Fig 2–4).

When the thrombus occludes the IVC, the extent of propagation up the IVC toward the liver, diaphragm, or heart cannot be determined from a study done only from below (Fig 5–5). A transbrachial, transatrial contrast study is then needed to study the atrium and upper aspect of the IVC. The risk is low, although we have seen one case of a fatal preoperative, noncancerous, saddle pulmonary embolus in a patient with a tumor thrombus in the atrium occurring 1 week after this study. The potential of either benign or malignant embolic events or acute proximal propagation of the thrombus has prompted Skinner et al[12] to advise the administration of IV heparin while awaiting surgery.

In our experience CT scans and ultrasound examinations have not been sufficiently accurate in defining the distal extent of the thrombus to justify sole reliance on these studies. Some authors have had better results. Magnetic resonance imaging, however, may be precise in imaging the thrombus and may obviate the need for other studies. The ability to visualize the thrombus in both coronal and transverse views with multiple techniques is helpful (Fig 5–6).

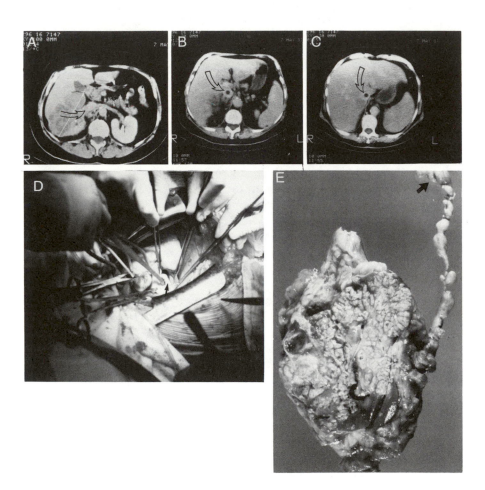

FIG 5–2.
Difficulty in defining upper extent of IVC tumor thrombus. **A,** CT scan demonstrates large RCC in right kidney with associated extension into IVC (*arrow*). **B,** IVC tumor thrombus seen as circular filling defect in the cava in the middle portion of the intrahepatic cava (*arrow*). **C,** filling defect persists into the upper portion of the intrahepatic cava (*arrow*). **D,** intraoperative photograph through right atriotomy. *Arrow* shows distal end of tumor thrombus protruding into the atrial lumen. **E,** right renal tumor bivalved demonstrates the lobulated tumor thrombus that extends up into the atrium. The tiny diameter and friability of the tumor thrombus makes intraoperative embolization a strong possibility. *Black arrow* shows segment of thrombus protruding into atrium. Patient is free of disease at 14 months after operation.

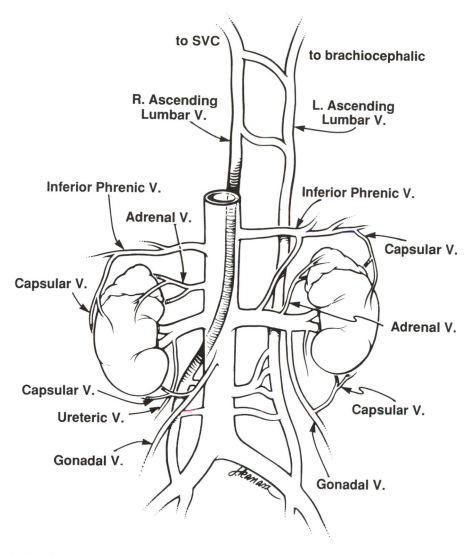

FIG 5–3.
Normal collateral circulation of right and left renal veins. (From Clayman RV, Gonzalez R, Fraley EE: *J Urol* 1980; 123:157–163. Used by permission.)

Ensuring that the thrombus that extends to the diaphragm does not extend into the atrium has been occasionally difficult. Although every study is not needed in every patient with a large tumor thrombus, one must be confident in the data available, and if there is any doubt, more information is needed.

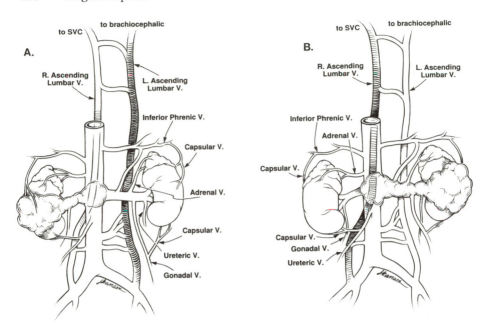

FIG 5–4.
Hypertrophy of collateral venous circulation caused by either right-sided (**A**) or left-sided (**B**) renal tumor. (From Clayman RV, Gonzalez R, Fraley EE: *J Urol* 1980; 123:157–163. Used by permission.)

JUDGING OPERABILITY

Although we can technically remove an RCC with an IVC thrombus, judgment is necessary relative to the wisdom of operating on any particular patient. In the past many patients underwent nephrectomy and thrombectomy even with nonresectable distant metastases with the idea of inducing a regression by removal of the primary lesion. Regression of metastases after nephrectomy, however, is a rare event, occurring in much less than 1% of cases, and must be contrasted with an operative mortality in this type of patient of 4% to 5% at best.[13] As data became available from Cleveland Clinic Foundation and other institutions, it became clear that patients who had preexisting metastases and an IVC thrombus had an extremely poor prognosis, and few patients lived beyond 1 year with or without surgery.[7, 9, 14–18] Thus surgery of this magnitude may not be justifiable unless palliation is definitely necessary or an effective systemic therapy becomes available.

On the basis of this reasoning, we do a more exhaustive search for metastases in a patient with an IVC thrombus than we do with a lower stage RCC. The risk of metastases is higher, thus more abnormalities are found. A chest x-ray film and usually a chest and abdominal CT scan are done. A bone scan and a head CT scan are not routinely obtained with RCC patients without symptoms but are done in patients with a large IVC thrombus.

Currently, we believe that grossly enlarged lymph nodes with metastases make attempts at resection ill-advised. Occasionally, hyperplastic lymph nodes can be quite large, and aspiration biopsy of a node may confirm metastases, and a laparotomy can be avoided. We are reluctant to declare a patient's condition inoperable purely on the basis of a CT finding of enlarged lymph nodes unless the growth is extremely characteristic of a malignant pattern. Even in this setting, biopsy is wise to ensure that a lymphoma or another type of malignancy is not present.

In an elderly patient who has a large thrombus and in whom cardiac bypass will be needed, coronary arteriography can be valuable in defining the potential risk of bypass. At Cleveland Clinic Foundation 25 patients with RCC had cardiac bypass to assist in tumor thrombus removal. A concurrent coronary artery bypass

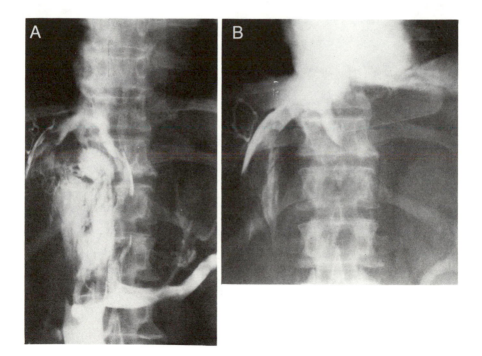

FIG 5–5.
A, near complete occlusion of IVC resulting from IVC tumor thrombus extending up to the level of the diaphragm identified on contrast injection from below. **B,** transatrial contrast injection of right atrium demonstrates uppermost extent of the tumor at the level of the diaphragm.

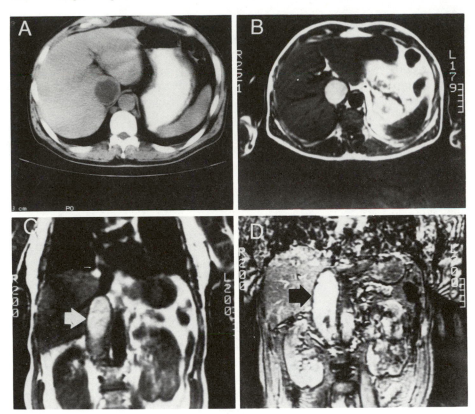

FIG 5–6.
Intrahepatic IVC tumor thrombus imaged by several techniques. **A,** CT scan demonstrates intrahepatic tumor thrombus with near complete occlusion and enlargement of the cava. **B,** T_1 weighted transverse magnetic resonance image at same level. **C,** T_1 weighted coronal magnetic resonance image demonstrates tumor thrombus (*arrow*) to level of uppermost hepatic veins. **D,** coronal magnetic resonance image at same level (*arrow*) with proton density image with flip angle at 15 degrees. This particular imaging technique is sensitive to changes in blood flow.

to the left anterior descending coronary artery because of high grade stenosis has been done in three patients to lessen the risk of a lethal perioperative myocardial infarction.

OPERATIVE TECHNIQUE

As stated earlier, the operative technique is dictated by the level of the thrombus. Incisions that can be used are a transverse bilateral subcostal (Chevron), midline (with or without a median sternotomy), or a high thoracoabdominal incision (Fig 5–7). For level I or II lesions we most commonly use a transperitoneal transverse incision unless the tumor in the kidney is a large upper pole mass. A right thoracoabdominal incision gives excellent exposure, but it takes longer and can expose the patient to potential additional complications.

Some authors[12] advocate a thoracoabdominal approach in essentially all cases. For right-sided tumors the incision is extended inferiorly in the midline (Fig 5–8). For left-sided tumors the same incision is used, but additional extension to the left subcostal area is included to provide better exposure in the left upper quadrant.

A self-retaining retractor fixed to the table has been extremely helpful in providing constant, untiring exposure for difficult renal surgery. A Bookwalter retractor is ideal in our experience (Fig 5–9).

Collateral veins associated with IVC obstruction are often the first problem encountered in the case. The vessels are often large, thin walled, friable, and must be patiently controlled throughout the dissection. Mobilization of the colon or duodenum done quickly in a standard radical nephrectomy can be tedious

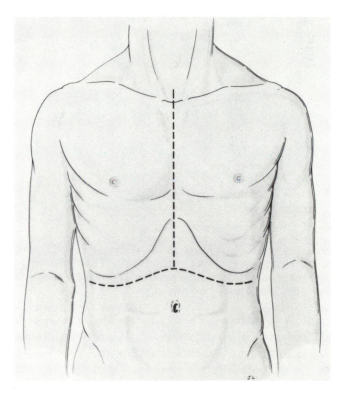

FIG 5–7.
Bilateral transverse upper abdominal incision used for nephrectomy, occasionally combined if necessary with median sternotomy. (From Novick AC, Montie JE: Surgery for renal cell carcinoma involving the inferior vena cava, in Novick AC, Streem SS, Pontes JE [eds]: *Stewart's Operative Urology.* Baltimore, Williams & Wilkins Co, 1989. Used by permission.)

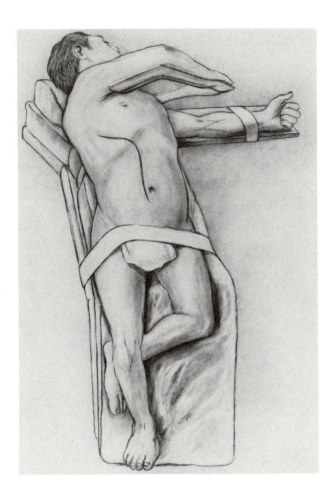

FIG 5–8.
Right thoracoabdominal excision for right-sided tumor. (From Skinner DG, Lieskovsky G, Pritchett TR: Management of renal cell carcinoma involving the vena cava, in Skinner DG, Lieskovski G [eds]: *Diagnosis and Management of Genitourinary Cancer.* Philadelphia, WB Saunders Company, 1988, pp 697, 699. Used by permission.)

in this setting. Early ligation of the renal artery to lessen pressure in the venous system is desirable but can be difficult as well because of distortion from the primary tumor, a fibrotic reaction present around the occluded IVC, or reactive lymph nodes. For right-sided carcinomas, ligation of the right renal artery between the aorta and IVC is helpful. The origin of the right renal artery is consistently just inferior to the left renal vein as it enters the IVC (Fig 5–10). If the left renal vein is retracted superiorly, the right renal artery can be identified immediately after it leaves the aorta. It is not necessary to divide the artery at this stage, but double ligation now allows the artery to be divided later in the case when better exposure is available. Ligation of the renal artery must be done with little traction on the IVC when a small friable thrombus is present.

Although preoperative angioinfarction might be an advantage in this particular part of the procedure, we have rarely used it because of its own inherent disadvantages of pain and potential complications. Angioinfarction can sometimes decrease the size of the arterialized IVC thrombus if one waits a few weeks to do the operation, but only anecdotal observations are available.

For a level I or II thrombus, dissection proceeds around the involved renal vein and IVC. Because of the potential for dislodgment of the small thrombus with mobilization of the kidney, it is good to obtain control of the IVC above the thrombus with a Rumel tourniquet that may or may not be completely tightened. Complete occlusion of the IVC above a nonobstructing thrombus often causes hypotension and can lead to increased venous pressure in many of the collateral veins and magnify bleeding from these veins. Vascular control is also obtained from the contralateral renal vein and lower IVC.

Several potential sites of bleeding are evident during dissection of the renal vein or IVC. The most common problem is the lumbar vein entering the posterior aspect of the left renal vein slightly lateral to the aorta (Fig 5–11). This vein usually needs to be doubly ligated and divided to allow good exposure to get to the left renal artery. Unfortunately, if control of the lumbar side of the vein

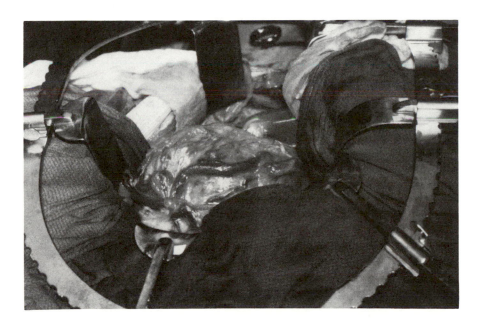

FIG 5–9.
Bookwalter self-retaining retractor is extremely useful for providing constant, untiring exposure of the retroperitoneum.

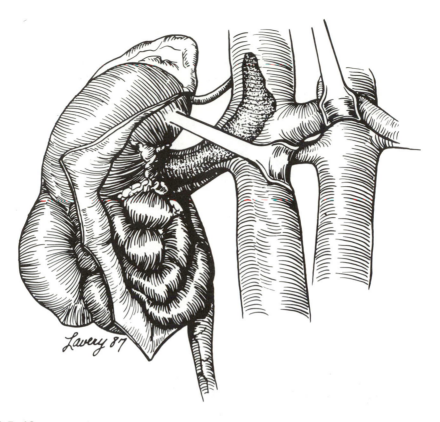

FIG 5–10.
The origin of the right renal artery behind the vena cava at the level of the entrance of the left renal vein. (From Novick AC, Montie JE: Surgery for renal cell carcinoma involving the inferior vena cava, in Novick AC, Streem SS, Pontes JE [eds]: *Stewart's Operative Urology.* Baltimore, Williams and Wilkins Co, 1989. Used by permission.)

is lost, the stump may retract into the paraspinus muscles; deep suture ligatures may be necessary to provide hemostasis. Similarly, the left adrenal vein, the right gonadal vein, and the lumbar vein entering the posterior aspect of the IVC at the level of the renal hilum may cause troublesome bleeding if not adequately controlled. The right adrenal vein poses a particular problem because it enters the posterolateral aspect of the IVC at the superior margin of the right adrenal gland, and exposure here may be difficult.

Level I

A level I thrombus (<2 cm into the IVC) requires adequate exposure of the right ventricle and IVC. After the renal artery is ligated, an angled or curved Satinsky clamp is placed on the IVC, ideally so that it does not completely occlude the IVC (Fig 5–12). The clamp remains in place until the rest of the kidney is mobilized, and then the ostia of the right ventricle into the IVC is opened and the thrombus is removed. "Milking" the thrombus back into the renal vein can occasionally be helpful. An alternate approach is to divide the renal vein, wrap the exposed thrombus in the right ventricle with gauze to minimize tumor spill, and reconstruct the IVC at this time before mobilization of the kidney. The cavotomy is closed with a running 4–0 or 5–0 vascular suture (Fig 5–13).

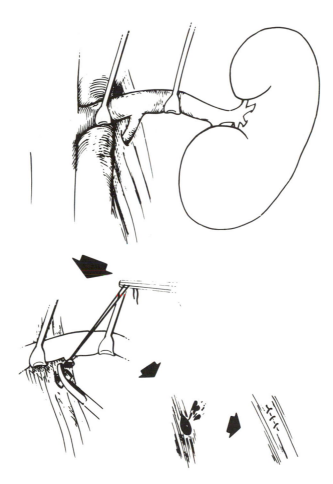

FIG 5–11.
Entrance of lumbar vein into the posterior aspect of the left renal vein, slightly lateral to the aorta. (From Novick AC, Montie JE: Surgery for renal cell carcinoma involving the inferior vena cava, in Novick AC, Streem SS, Pontes JE [eds]: *Stewart's Operative Urology.* Baltimore, Williams and Wilkins Co, 1989. Used by permission.)

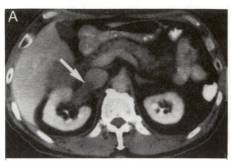
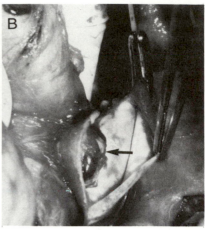

FIG 5–12.
Level I tumor thrombus. **A,** CT scan demonstrates tumor thrombus protruding into the vena cava at the level of the renal ostia. **B,** intraoperative photograph shows Satinsky clamp partially occluding IVC, anterolateral vena cavotomy at the site of the right renal vein ostia, and *arrow* demonstrating tumor thrombus at level of renal vein ostia.

Level II

With a level II thrombus the IVC must be completely occluded below the hepatic veins to allow extraction. Some degree of hypotension may result from this but usually is manageable with volume expansion. To allow placement of a vascular clamp sufficiently high on the IVC so as to be above the thrombus, small veins from the caudate lobe of the liver frequently need to be divided. These may be short and must be carefully controlled with suture ligature. After complete venous control is obtained, a cavotomy is made at the entrance of the involved renal vein into the IVC. A level II thrombus usually extracts easily, and the cavotomy is then closed (Fig 5–14).

Some authors have advised that for a left-sided tumor it is wiser to occlude the right renal artery rather than the right renal vein. Our experience has not demonstrated such a need or particular advantage.

Level III

A level III lesion implies that there is a thrombus in the main intrahepatic portion of the IVC, such that a clamp cannot be placed above the thrombus but below the main hepatic veins. Earlier published descriptions of techniques advised the use of a Foley catheter to extract the thrombus through a cavotomy followed by immediate application of a vascular clamp on the IVC.[19] The "substantial gush of venous blood" accompanying the removal of the tumor thrombus is believed to be helpful in flushing out a small particulate tumor.[19] When the thrombus came out in one piece and the clamp happened to be applied in the exact right spot on the IVC, the procedure was quite straightforward. Disastrous consequences followed, however, if the thrombus was fragmented or the clamp not applied precisely because of poor exposure resulting from bleeding. In our opinion this technique is unpredictable and exposes the patient to considerable risk. Two approaches are now possible that allow the resection to be done in a more controlled situation.

One approach requires control of the intrapericardial IVC, porta hepatis (Pringle's maneuver), superior mesenteric artery, inferior mesenteric artery, lower IVC, contralateral right ventricle, and lumbar veins as needed (Fig 5–15). The approach recommended by Skinner et al[12] is through a right thoracoab-

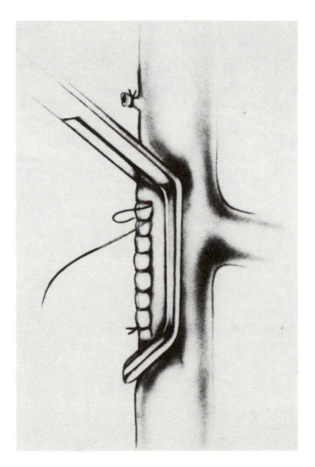

FIG 5–13.
Closure of a cavotomy with running suture. Good exposure allows closure to avoid sutures that take too large of a "bite" on the IVC and thus narrow the lumen.

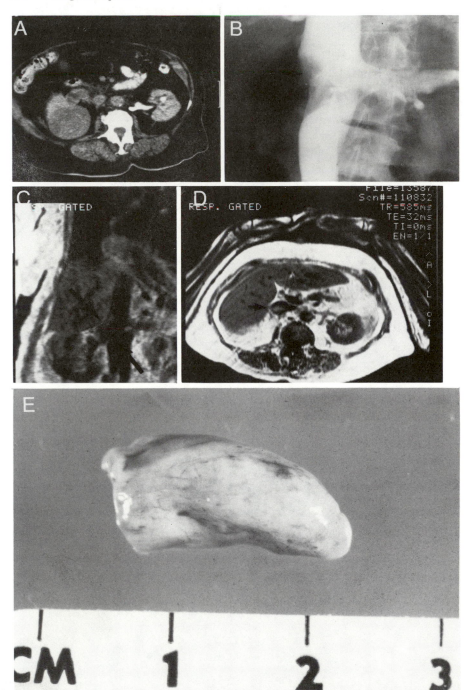

FIG 5–14.
Level II thrombus. **A,** CT scan demonstrates right RCC with apparent thrombus in IVC. **B,** inferior venacavography. *Arrow* points to filling defect corresponding with level II thrombus. **C,** coronal magnetic resonance image. *Arrows* demonstrate thrombus protruding into IVC. **D,** transverse magnetic resonance image of infrahepatic IVC. *Arrow* shows tumor thrombus in lumen. **E,** gross photograph of distal portion of tumor thrombus corresponding to the filling defect seen in **D**.

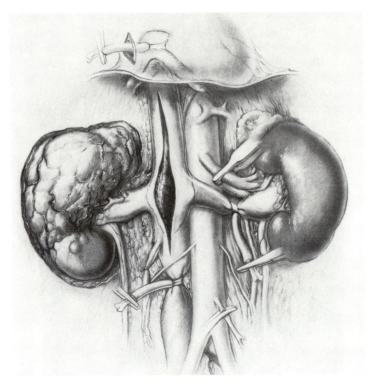

FIG 5–15.
Elements of vascular control with Rumel tourniquets needed for excision of intrahepatic tumor thrombus. Pringle's maneuver (occluding porta hepatis) is not shown. (From Skinner DG, Lieskovsky G, Pritchett TR: Management of renal cell carcinoma involving the vena cava, in Skinner DG, Lieskovsky G [eds]: *Diagnosis and Management of Genitourinary Cancer.* Philadelphia, WB Saunders Company, 1988. Used by permission.)

dominal incision resecting rib 8. The liver is rotated medially to expose the anterolateral surface of the intrahepatic IVC. The primary advantage of this procedure is that cardiac bypass and systemic heparinization are avoided. The disadvantage is that the porta hepatis can be occluded for only 15 to 20 minutes; hypotension may be a problem with the upper IVC and porta hepatis occluded, and back bleeding from posterior lumbar vessels that might not be divided may be brisk. If the thrombus is bulky and adherent to the IVC, removal of the thrombus and closure of a long cavotomy might require more than 20 minutes. Good results have been obtained with experienced surgeons; we believe that this approach is most appropriate for the thrombus that is likely to be extracted intact easily (Fig 5–16).

Venous bypass has been advocated as an adjunct with the goal of reducing hypotension.[20] Blood is drained from the IVC below the thrombus and returned to the right atrium by means of a centrifugal venous pump. Although somewhat simpler than cardiac bypass, systemic heparinization is still necessary.

The alternate approach to a level III lesion is the use of cardiac bypass, with or without circulatory arrest, generally through a transverse incision combined with a median sternotomy. The use of cardiac bypass to assist in the resection of RCC was reported by Marshall et al[21] as early as 1970. Since then, individual cases or small series of cases have been described with acceptable results. Turini et al[22] stated in 1986 that fewer than 30 cases had been reported. Undoubtedly more cases had been attempted but were unsuccessful and thus not reported. The Cleveland Clinic now has experience in 26 cases with the use of cardiac

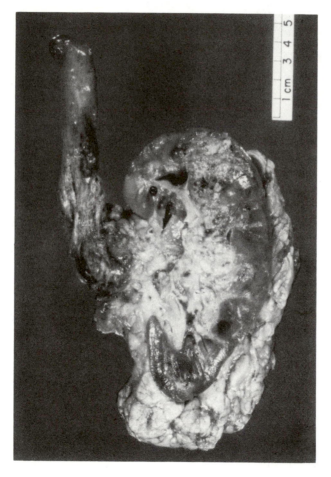

FIG 5–16.
Operative photograph of right-sided renal tumor demonstrates ideal level III thrombus, which extracts easily without adherence to IVC wall.

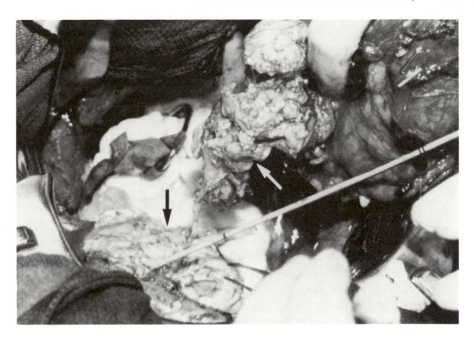

FIG 5–17.
Intraoperative photograph demonstrates removal of large level III thrombus (same case as presented in Fig 5–4). Fragmentation of the necrotic thrombus is evident, and a portion of the tumor thrombus remains intact with the kidney (*white arrow*). The "cheesy" thrombus adherent to the IVC wall is demonstrated by the *black arrow*. An attempt had been made to extract the thrombus intact with a venous 45 ml balloon catheter.

bypass. Cardiac bypass by itself for coronary artery disease is one of the most common operations performed in the United States, and the mortality for isolated single vessel coronary artery disease is approximately 1%. The main advantage of cardiac bypass is the control afforded; massive, sudden bleeding is reliably prevented. The disadvantage is the need for systemic heparinization while the patient is on bypass. It is extremely important to mobilize the entire kidney and obtain absolute hemostasis before initiating bypass.

Extraction of an adherent thrombus with either method requires patience and persistence. Frank invasion of the wall of the IVC does not need to be present for the thrombus to be attached to the wall (Fig 5–17). An endarterectomy knife, tonsil clamp, or blunt forceps have been used to strip away fragments. Logic predicts that this type of lesion would be associated with a worse prognosis, but experience is too small to draw conclusions.[9, 14–18] Frank invasion of the IVC wall requiring resection has been associated with a worse prognosis, but this is also an observation based on small numbers of patients and was not confirmed in the recent Cleveland Clinic Foundation series.[8]

Level IV

The presence of tumor thrombus above the diaphragm indicates the need for cardiac bypass as an adjunct. Isolated successful cases of extraction of the thrombus from below have been reported; however, the potential to underestimate the extent of the thrombus with lesions at the level of the diaphragm, even with all modalities, is real, and bypass offers the flexibility to deal with any situation that may become evident.[16, 18]

Cardiac Bypass

The traditional method of resecting a level IV thrombus requires collaboration with a cardiothoracic surgical team including the surgeon, anesthesiologist, and pump team. In published articles it has been stated that the cardiac surgery team is on "standby." In reality, this should require that the procedure be performed in an operating room commonly used for open heart surgery with all the necessary support services available. The pump oxygenator must be in the room. Preparations less than this are likely to be inadequate because recruitment of the cardiothoracic team into the operating room implies that the thrombus is more extensive than appreciated preoperatively or that bleeding or loss of control of the thrombus has occurred, and time will be of the essence. To schedule such a case in a standard urology operating room with the expectation of a cardiothoracic team helping if something goes wrong invites chaos.

The first step in using cardiac bypass requires complete mobilization of the kidney until it is attached only by the involved renal vein. The IVC, lumbar veins, and contralateral renal vein are controlled. After hemostasis is complete, a median sternotomy is performed and the right atrium and aorta are cannulated. Cannulation of the femoral vessels has been abandoned in recent years because collateral venous return from the lower half of the body is usually already developed. Control of potential sources of venous bleeding should be obtained to minimize bleeding from the cavotomy. The patient is given heparin, and bypass is initiated. After the IVC is opened, the "pump" sucker is used to collect and recycle blood through the pump. A 25 μm filter that only allows single cells to be recirculated is used. A theoretic risk of returning individual cancer cells to the circulation exists, but the true hazard of this is unknown. Occasionally exposure can be obscured by back bleeding, but support of the cardiovascular system is not a concern.

The cavotomy must be large enough to remove the thrombus; in cases in which the cava is three to four times normal size, a large (i.e., 15 cm) cavotomy may be necessary (Fig 5–18). Manual traction on the kidney and thrombus, with the help of a 45 ml venous Fogarty balloon catheter placed up the IVC into the atrium, usually extracts the thrombus (Fig 5–19). Often the cardiothoracic surgeon can help by pushing the thrombus inferiorly through an atriotomy (Fig 5–20). Occasionally the thrombus is "dumbbell" shaped, and the widened intraatrial segment needs to be removed through the atrium. After the thrombus

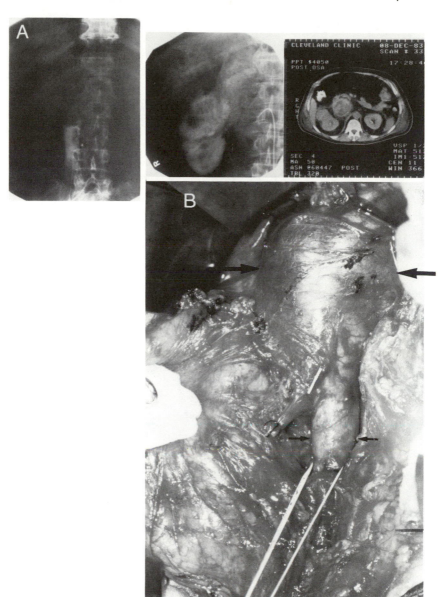

FIG 5–18.
A, inferior venacavogram, angiogram, and CT scan of intrahepatic IVC demonstrate occluded vena cava with tumor thrombus enlarging IVC to 3 to 4 times normal size. **B,** intraoperative photograph with *small arrows* that define normal caliber IVC in the infrarenal region and *large arrows* that define the diameter of markedly enlarged IVC caused by tumor thrombus.

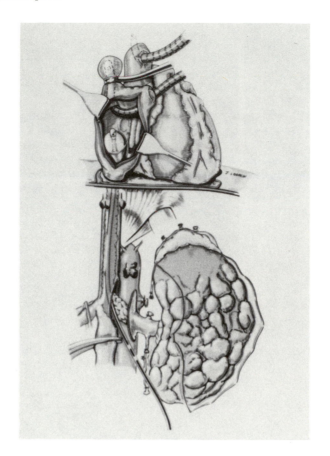

FIG 5–19.
A 45 ml venous Fogarty balloon catheter is placed above the level of the thrombus (into the atrium if necessary) through a cavotomy and used to assist in manual traction inferiorly to remove the thrombus. (From Novick AC, Montie JE: Surgery for renal cell carcinoma involving the inferior vena cava, in Novick AC, Streem SS, Pontes JE [eds]: *Stewart's Operative Urology.* Baltimore, Williams and Wilkins Co, 1989. Used by permission.)

has been removed, vascular clamps can be applied to stop back bleeding and improve exposure, allowing the cavotomy to be closed. Bypass is terminated, the patient decannulated, and the heparin is reversed.

Circulatory Arrest

Circulatory arrest is an adjunct to cardiac bypass. Profound hypothermia (18° to 20° C core temperature) allows all circulation to be interrupted and 95% of the patient's blood volume to be drained out of the body into the bypass machine. There is no blood flow to any organ. This allows any operation to be performed in an entirely bloodless field with unsurpassed exposure.

Circulatory arrest has been used for many years for the repair of complicated congenital heart defects. The technique has been used infrequently in adults, primarily in cases of large thoracic aortic aneurysms. In 1984, Marshall et al[23] and Krane et al[24] reported single cases of the successful use of the technique for the resection of a large RCC thrombus with IVC extension into the atrium. Since then, additional experience has been reported from the Cleveland Clinic and from Johns Hopkins Hospital.[18, 25] Our experience now includes 23 cases with two operative deaths (9%). Three additional patients had prolonged recovery (>30 days of hospitalization), but most of the patients have done remarkably well with a median postoperative hospital stay of 9 days.

The expertise of a cardiothoracic anesthesiology team experienced in the use of circulatory arrest is a necessity. Complications directly attributable to circulatory arrest have not been seen; specifically, there has been no apparent neurologic damage and no significant hepatic or renal dysfunction. The greatest concern is the potential for coagulopathy associated with bypass and circulatory

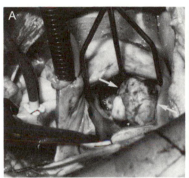
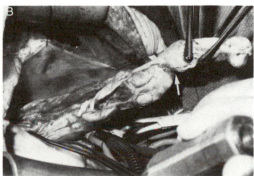
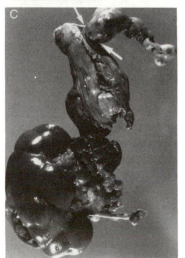

FIG 5–20.
Level IV thrombus. **A,** intraoperative photograph through right atriotomy demonstrates large tumor thrombus occupying most of the right atrium. **B,** intraoperative photograph demonstrates extraction of the tumor thrombus through the right atriotomy. Thrombus to the right of the *arrow* is the intraatrial segment. **C,** gross photograph of tumor thrombus and removed kidney. Thrombus to the right of the *arrows* is the intraatrial segment. Part of the distal portion of this thrombus would periodically prolapse through the tricuspid valve causing an arrhythmia. It is now 50 months after the operation, and the patient remains free of disease.

arrest. After a standard cardiac bypass procedure, a postoperative coagulopathy is seen in approximately 3% of cases. The addition of profound hypothermia will increase the potential for platelet dysfunction, but the frequency of a clinically significant abnormality is unknown. In our first 22 patients, three patients (14%) needed another operation for bleeding within the first 24 hours, and all recovered. Several other patients had abnormal coagulation measurements that resolved without clinically significant bleeding. This coagulopathy is the greatest threat to the patient undergoing this procedure and will probably limit the application of circulatory arrest.

When circulatory arrest is added to the operative technique, extraction of the thrombus is easy (see Fig 5–20). There is no need to rush because circulatory arrest can be used safely for approximately 60 minutes. Dissection of the IVC, often difficult with a large thrombus in multiple collateral veins, is only needed to allow closure of the cavotomy. One can be sure all tumor fragments are removed. A 10 to 15 cm cavotomy is easily closed. A key element for success is a cardiothoracic team experienced with the use of profound hypothermia. We have employed use of circulatory arrest for large level III lesions and for level IV tumors.

RESULTS

Postoperative Complications

Radical nephrectomy with IVC thrombectomy has all the risks of a radical nephrectomy alone, with the additional difficulties associated with vascular aspects of the procedure. Tumors with an IVC thrombus are likely to be larger lesions, also making the operation harder. The operative mortality accumulated from several series in the past 10 years is listed in Table 5–2. The higher rates of greater than 10% were often based on earlier experience; more recent series are reporting mortality in the range of 4% to 10%.

TABLE 5–2.
Operative Mortality for Radical Nephrectomy and IVC
Tumor Thrombectomy for RCC

Author (yr)	Percent	No. of Patients
Abdelsayed (1978)[26]	9	1/11
Schefft (1978)[7]	14	3/21
Kearney (1981)[14]	4	1/25
Cherrie (1982)[15]	11	3/27
Sogani (1983)[27]	6	1/16
Sosa (1984)[28]	16	4/24
Pritchett (1986)[16]	12	3/25
Neves (1987)[9]	9	5/54
O'Donahoe (1987)[29]	10	1/10
Libertino (1987)[17]	4	2/44
Bintz (1988)[30]	8	1/12
Montie (1988)[8]	4	2/48
	Total	9% (27/317)

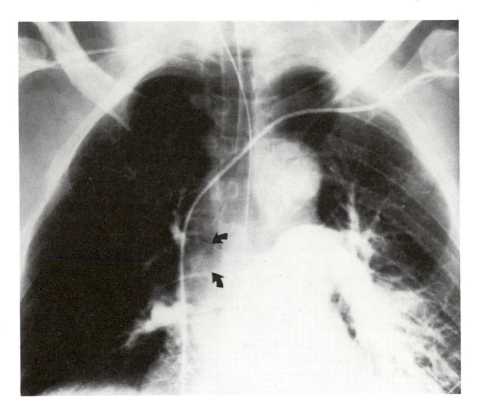

FIG 5–21.
Pulmonary angiogram demonstrates complete occlusion of the right pulmonary artery (*arrows*) from a saddle embolus composed of tumor thrombus from a level II IVC tumor thrombus.

An intraoperative tumor embolization to the lungs is usually a fatal complication. Only a small number of cases are described in the literature; successful extraction from the pulmonary artery has been reported in children and in one case from Cleveland Clinic Foundation. In our series of 48 cases, there was one intraoperative embolus that actually was difficult to diagnose. Despite embolectomy at 48 hours after operation, the patient died (Fig 5–21). Clearly prevention is a necessity. Vena cava clips have been recommended to help avoid this complication.[27]

Renal failure is a concern because of the potential need to (1) temporarily occlude venous drainage of the remaining kidney, (2) compromise venous drainage as a result of a narrowed IVC after reconstruction, or (3) compromise venous drainage by resection of the IVC and ligation of the remaining renal vein.

In the Cleveland Clinic Foundation series the only patient needing dialysis was one rendered anephric by the operation. Other series[14, 17] report a 0% to 25% need for dialysis. Our view is that the use of cardiac bypass with circulatory arrest has been helpful in preventing intraoperative renal ischemia.

Ligation of the left renal vein near the IVC with a right RCC is usually safe because of collateral circulation available through the left adrenal, gonadal, and lumbar veins. This step is usually only needed when the cava is resected entirely because of a large thrombus invading the wall. With a thrombus this size there is usually preexisting complete occlusion of the IVC, thus the collateral drainage has had time to expand. Ligation of the right renal vein with a left RCC is rarely feasible because the potential for collateral circulation is less. We have done so successfully in one case. In the rare situation in which the right renal venous drainage cannot be maintained, autotransplantation to the pelvis or a venous graft from the renal vein to the portal vein is a potential option.[2]

It is striking that venous complications in the preoperative or postoperative period are not seen more often. This is a consequence of the insidious growth of the thrombus, allowing collateral veins through the azygous system to expand.

Proximal propagation of the thrombus into the lower IVC and iliac veins is usually benign but can be long-standing and impossible to remove even under direct vision at surgery as a result of fibrous reaction and organization of the thrombus. If all thrombus or clot cannot be extracted from the IVC, the IVC should probably be ligated or clipped to prevent postoperative pulmonary emboli.[9]

Postoperative thrombosis of the IVC or pulmonary emboli resulting from a narrowed IVC after partial IVC resection is uncommon. Routine heparinization or long-term anticoagulation has not been used in the uncomplicated case but may be warranted if the IVC is narrowed substantially. Silent occlusion postoperatively of the IVC may be more common than appreciated and may be clinically undetected. A systematic study of all postoperative patients with either magnetic resonance imaging or an inferior venacavogram has not been done.

Survival

The most important variable relative to long-term survival with resection of an IVC thrombus is the presence or absence of metastases identified preoperatively (Fig 5–22). Few patients with metastases survive more than 1 year with or without surgery. An increasingly frequent dilemma will involve the participation of patients in investigative trials with BRMs such as tumor-infiltrating lymphocytes or autologous vaccines that require tumor material for the treatment (see Chapter 7). In addition, most BRM trials to date have suggested a higher probability for a favorable response if a bulky primary tumor is absent. Thus more pressure will be exerted to remove the primary tumor in the kidney with the anticipation of patient participation in a well defined and closely controlled clinical trial. Certainly patients will be selected for a good performance status, a relatively small burden of metastatic disease, and good general health.

The 5-year survival after surgery in patients without metastases ranges from 20% to 50%, depending on patient selection in the individual series. The bottom line is that in the absence of any other effective treatment and the likelihood of morbidity from the thrombus, tumor resection can be recommended even though the long-term outlook may be poor. Many authors have looked for characteristics that might allow better stratification of the risk for relapse. Level of the thrombus has been believed to be a key variable by Sosa et al,[28] Pritchett et al,[16] and in the Cleveland Clinic Foundation series.[8] Other series from Cherrie et al,[15] Libertino et al,[17] and O'Donohoe et al[29] have confirmed this observation.

A recent Cleveland Clinic Foundation review analyzed 48 patients undergoing resection of an IVC thrombus from RCC. In patients without metastases several variables were examined relative to actuarial survival, analyzed by the Log Rank test.[31, 32] Lymph node status (p = 0.75, Fig 5–23, A), perinephric fat invasion (p = 0.33, Fig 5–23, B), resection of the IVC (p = 0.47, Fig 5–23, C), and intact or piecemeal resection (p = 0.90, Fig 5–23, D) were examined and found to be statistically insignificant predictors.

Noteworthy is the observation that atrial extension was associated with a significantly worse survival than either renal infrahepatic or intrahepatic disease (p = 0.005, Fig 5–23, E). It is difficult to find survivors for greater than 5 years documented in the literature. This must be considered a preliminary conclusion because fewer than 50 surgically successful cases (nine from Cleveland Clinic Foundation) have been reported.

Unfortunately, the relatively small number of cases of IVC tumor thrombus available from any one institution and the inability to collate data from several series have not allowed the necessary multivariate analyses to be performed.

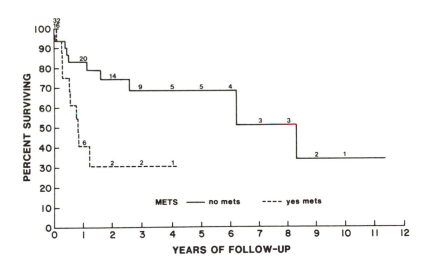

FIG 5–22.
Actuarial survival estimated by Kaplan-Meier Curve comparing patients with metastases identified before surgery and those without metastases. Difference between curves by Log Rank test showed p = 0.01.

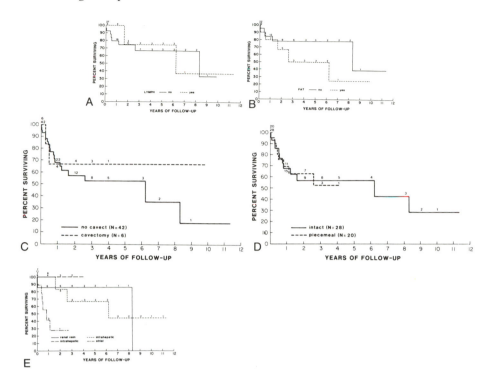

FIG 5–23.
A, actuarial survival for patients with no metastases relative to lymph node metastases. **B,** actuarial survival for patients with no metastases relative to perinephric fat involvement. **C,** actuarial survival for patients with no metastases relative to cavotomy or cavectomy. **D,** actuarial survival for patients with no metastases relative to thrombectomy removal intact or piecemeal. **E,** actuarial survival for patients without metastases relative to the level of the IVC thrombus.

In summary, RCC with an IVC thrombus is part of the spectrum of advanced local growth. Logically the prognosis will be a reflection of this. Advances in the surgical techniques needed for removal allow a more aggressive treatment, but additional experience is needed to judge the wisdom of this approach in the long term.

REFERENCES

1. McDonald JR, Priestly JT: Malignant tumors of the kidney; surgical and prognostic significance of tumor thrombosis of the renal vein. *Surg, Gynecol, Obstet* 1943; 77:295–306.
2. Berg AA: Malignant hypernephroma of the kidney. Its clinical course and diagnosis, with a description of the author's method of radical operative cure. *Surg, Gynecol, Obstet* 1913; 17:463–471.
3. Judd ES, Scoll AJ: Thrombosis and embolism resulting from renal tumors. *JAMA* 1924; 82:75–78.

4. Robson CJ, Churchill BM, Anderson W: The results of radical nephrectomy for renal cell carcinoma. *J Urol* 1969; 101:297–301.
5. Skinner DG, Pfister RF, Colvin R: Extension of renal cell carcinoma into the vena cava: The rationale for aggressive surgical management. *J Urol* 1972; 107:711–716.
6. Komatsu H, Yoh T, Murakami K, et al: Renal cell carcinoma with intracaval tumor thrombus extending to the diaphragm: Ultrasonography and surgical management. *J Urol* 1985; 134:122–125.
7. Schefft P, Novick AC, Straffon RA, et al: Surgery for renal cell carcinoma extending into the inferior vena cava. *J Urol* 1978; 120:28–31.
8. Montie JE, El Ammar R, Pontes JE, et al: Renal cell carcinoma with inferior vena cava tumor thrombus. *J Urol* Submitted for publication.
9. Neves RJ, Zincke H: Surgical treatment of renal cancer with vena cava extension. *Br J Urol* 1987; 59:390–395.
10. Hedderich GS, O'Connor RJ, Reid EC, et al: Caval tumor thrombus complicating renal cell carcinoma: A surgical challenge. *Surgery* 1987; 102:614–620.
11. Siminovitch JMP, Montie JE, Straffon RA: Inferior venacavography in the preoperative assessment of renal adenocarcinoma. *J Urol* 1982; 128:908–909.
12. Skinner DG, Lieskovsky G, Pritchett TR: Management of renal cell carcinoma involving the vena cava, in Skinner DG, Lieskovsky G (eds): *Diagnosis and Management of Genitourinary Cancer.* Philadelphia, WB Saunders Company, 1988.
13. Montie JE, Stewart BH, Straffon RA, et al: The role of adjunctive nephrectomy in patients with metastatic renal cell carcinoma. *J Urol* 1977; 117:272–275.
14. Kearney GP, Waters WB, Klein LA, et al: Results of inferior vena cava resection for renal cell carcinoma. *J Urol* 1981; 125:769–773.
15. Cherrie RJ, Goldman DG, Lindner A, et al: Prognostic implications of vena caval extension of renal cell carcinoma. *J Urol* 1982; 128:910–912.
16. Pritchett TR, Lieskovsky G, Skinner DG: Extension of renal cell carcinoma into the vena cava: Clinical review and surgical approach. *J Urol* 1986; 135:460–464.
17. Libertino JA, Zinman L, Watkins E, Jr: Long-term results of resection of renal cell cancer with extension into inferior vena cava. *J Urol* 1986; 137:21–24.
18. Marshall FF, Dietrick DD, Baumgartner WA, et al: Surgical management of renal cell carcinoma with intracaval neoplastic extension above the hepatic veins. *J Urol* 1988; 139:1166–1172.
19. Freed SZ, Gliedman ML: The removal of renal carcinoma thrombus extending into the right atrium. *J Urol* 1975; 113:163–165.
20. Attwood S, Lang DM, Goiti J, et al: Venous bypass for surgical resection of renal carcinoma invading the vena cava: A new approach. *Br J Urol* 1988; 61:402–405.
21. Marshall VF, Middleton RG, Holswade GR, et al: Surgery for renal cell carcinoma in the vena cava. *J Urol* 1970; 103:412–420.
22. Turini D, Selli C, Barbanti G, et al: Removal of renal cell carcinoma extending to the supradiaphragmatic vena cava with the aid of cardiopulmonary bypass. *Urol Int* 1986; 41:303–306.
23. Marshall FF, Reitz BA, Diamond DA: A new technique for management of renal cell carcinoma involving the right atrium: Hypothermia and cardiac arrest. *J Urol* 1984; 131:103–107.
24. Krane RJ, White RD, Davis Z, et al: Removal of renal cell carcinoma extending into the right atrium using cardiopulmonary bypass, profound hypothermia and circulatory arrest. *J Urol* 1984; 131:945–947.

25. Montie JE, Jackson CL, Cosgrove DM, et al: Resection of large inferior vena caval thrombi from renal cell carcinoma with the use of circulatory arrest. *J Urol* 1988; 139:25–28.
26. Abdelsayed MA, Bissada NK, Finkbeiner AE, et al: Renal tumors involving the inferior vena cava: Plan for management. *J Urol* 1978; 120:152–155.
27. Sogani PC, Herr HW, Bains MS, et al: Renal cell carcinoma extending into the inferior vena cava. *J Urol* 1983; 130:660–663.
28. Sosa RE, Muecke EC, Vaughn ED, et al: Renal cell carcinoma extending into the inferior vena cava: The prognostic significance of the level of vena caval involvement. *J Urol* 1984; 132:1097–1100.
29. O'Donohoe MK, Flanagan F, Fitzpatrick JM, et al: Surgical approach to inferior vena caval extension of renal carcinoma. *Br J Urol* 1987; 60:492–496.
30. Bintz M, Cogbill TH, Klein AS: Surgical treatment of renal cell carcinoma involving the inferior vena cava. *J Vasc Surg* 1987; 6:566–571.
31. Kaplan EL, Meier P: Nonparametric estimation from incomplete observations. *J Am Stat Assoc* 1958; 53:457–481.
32. Peto R, Pike ML, Armitage P, et al: Design and analysis of randomized clinical trials requiring prolonged observation of each patient. II. Analysis and examples. *Br J Cancer* 1977; 35:7–11.

6

The Problem of the Incidental Renal Mass

James E. Montie, M.D.

The widespread use of imaging studies of the upper abdomen has provided an interesting management dilemma in the form of the incidentally discovered renal mass. The mass is often small, and a radical nephrectomy seems excessive for a lesion that is not only asymptomatic but may not even be malignant. A historical perspective in this situation is valuable.

Before the era of CT and ultrasonography, the intravenous pyelogram (IVP) was the main radiologic procedure used to evaluate the kidneys. An IVP was rarely done in patients without urologic symptoms. In this setting occasionally a renal mass would be identified, commonly on a preoperative study before transurethral resection of the prostate for bladder outlet obstruction. By far the most common finding was a simple renal cyst, but it was not unusual for surgical exploration to be needed to establish the diagnosis.[1] Small lesions in the kidney, 2 to 3 cm in diameter, frequently would not be seen on the IVP.

The present circumstances are different. CT and ultrasonography are obtained for a variety of abdominal complaints, and the kidneys are often visualized incidentally.[2] CT and ultrasonography also facilitate identification of a 2 to 3 cm lesion. We thus have the dilemma of what to do with these lesions, since not all lesions are malignant, and the natural history of those that are malignant is not well defined.

Another opportunity for the detection of an asymptomatic renal mass is the general abdominal exploration at the time of a laparotomy.[3] The renal mass identified was previously "explored," occasionally with removal of the kidney, since that often was the ultimate means of establishing the diagnosis and treatment. Most of these lesions were cysts that can now be accurately confirmed by noninvasive imaging studies (see Chapter 2). Thus this "intraoperative consult" for the incidental renal mass requires clinical judgment and is discussed in more detail.[3]

TABLE 6–1.
Differential Diagnosis of Incidental
Renal Mass

1. Renal cyst, simple or complex
2. RCC
3. Oncocytoma
4. Adenoma
5. Angiomyolipoma
6. Other (rare)

DIFFERENTIAL DIAGNOSIS

The obvious concern with the incidentally discovered renal mass is RCC (Table 6–1). Simple renal cysts occur in approximately 25% of the population, and current imaging studies can confirm the diagnosis of a simple cyst in approximately 97% of cases (see Chapter 2).[4, 5] A complex cyst based on calcification, loculation, or inhomogeneous internal structures remains a diagnostic problem.

Most solid renal masses will be RCC. Renal adenomas are common in autopsy or pathology studies but usually are too small to be detected clinically.[6, 7]

The pathologic diagnosis of the entity of renal adenoma is debatable, as discussed in Chapter 2. Mukamel et al[8] reported a careful pathologic examination of kidneys removed for RCC. Renal adenomas were found in nine of 66 kidneys (14%), generally several millimeters in diameter and not larger than 1.5 cm. In the context of the discussion of the incidental renal mass and assuming renal adenomas are a definable benign entity, an argument could be made that an adenoma need not be removed if the diagnosis is firmly established. Given the uncertainty associated with establishing a firm diagnosis even when the whole specimen is available, however, it would be extraordinarily difficult for even an expert pathologist to make this diagnosis on the basis of an aspiration biopsy or a core biopsy.

An oncocytoma is a benign solid renal mass, often characterized by the absence of symptoms at the time of diagnosis. In an early review from Cleveland Clinic Foundation,[9] 10 of 11 cases were incidentally discovered renal masses. The natural history of oncocytoma is not truly known, but presumably observation would be safe because of the benign nature of the mass. Once again the problem is how one arrives at a reliable diagnosis, short of removal of the mass (see Chapter 2).

An angiomyolipoma can occasionally be seen in the absence of any symptoms. This, however, is a rare lesion, and unless the characteristic fat appearance is evident on a CT scan or magnetic resonance image, no distinction can be made from RCC preoperatively (see Chapter 2).

TREATMENT OPTIONS

Once an incidental renal mass has been identified, a logical evaluation plan is needed. If the mass has been identified in surgery at the time of another operation, the wisest approach is to proceed with the planned procedure and evaluate the mass postoperatively with traditional imaging studies (see Figure 2–16).[3] The temptation to "needle" the mass, unroof the cyst, perform a biopsy on the mass, or remove the entire kidney should be avoided. If the mass is a simple cyst, this can be confirmed easily with CT and ultrasonography with or without a percutaneous aspiration. If the mass is malignant, partial nephrectomy, total nephrectomy, or even no treatment may be viable options depending on the status of the contralateral kidney, other associated medical diseases, or the presence of metastases. The operative approach provided at the time of this initial procedure may not be ideal and could actually increase the overall risk. Informed consent from the patient for removal of all or part of the kidney also has not been possible obviously. Our philosophy has been that the safest approach is to have the appropriate information available before making a firm treatment decision, realizing that this might commit the patient to a second operation.[3]

If the incidental mass is discovered during CT or ultrasonography, further diagnostic studies are based on the level of suspicion for a malignancy. Simple cysts can be easily confirmed. Complex cysts or solid masses should be evaluated with a similar algorithm for sequential studies, as described in Chapter 2.

Once all needed imaging studies are available, we are left with whether an asymptomatic mass is likely to be an RCC or of undetermined disease. Options are as follows:

1. Observation only with repeat imaging studies in several months.
2. Percutaneous needle aspiration or core biopsy.
3. Surgical exploration with open biopsy.
4. Excisional biopsy with either enucleation or partial nephrectomy.
5. Radical nephrectomy.

Observation

Repeat evaluation in several months might be a wise approach in some patients. The natural history of some renal carcinomas may be protracted. If the patient is in poor general health and is asymptomatic, the risk of surgery may be more than the risk of delaying treatment to the cancer. Careful discussion with the patient and family is a key element in arriving at the proper decision.

Needle Aspiration and Biopsy

Needle biopsy or core biopsy may be valuable if a diagnosis of cancer is established. If a diagnosis of benign adenoma or oncocytoma is obtained, however, caution still needs to be exercised because of the inherent difficulties of sampling errors with the heterogeneity of the lesion, as discussed at length in Chapter 2. In a series by Juul et al[10] of 301 fine needle aspirates of solid renal masses, there were 25 (8%) false-negative studies. Seeding of the needle track is a theoretic risk and has been reported after biopsy with a large core needle (14 gauge), but this is extraordinarily rare.[11]

Our approach has been that because a biopsy with negative results will not obviate excision of the mass, the value is debatable. In the special circumstance of a patient in whom observation only is a strong consideration, aspiration biopsy may be helpful to indicate if this is a reasonable approach.

Excisional Biopsy With Enucleation or Partial Nephrectomy

For many circumstances with an incidentally discovered renal mass, excisional biopsy is an attractive approach (Figures 2–16 and 2–26). This is particularly well suited for the young patient, the small lesion (2 to 3 cm in diameter), or if there is any reason to preserve renal function (see Chapter 4). There is ample evidence to support partial nephrectomy as the sole treatment of the lesion even if it turns out to be malignant. If it is malignant, it is likely to be stage 1 (T_1 or T_2) and associated with a good prognosis (see Chapter 4). Although enucleation has been advised, the potential risk of leaving cancer cells in the fossa of the excised mass makes this an unattractive alternative.[12, 13]

Radical Nephrectomy

Proceeding directly to a radical nephrectomy in the case of a solid incidental renal mass would obviate many of the diagnostic questions. Although no clinical evidence documents an adverse effective removal of one kidney when the other kidney is entirely normal, it seems extreme to do this for what ultimately may be a benign lesion (see Chapter 4). Again, our philosophy is that larger lesions (>5 to 6 cm) are more likely to be malignant, less suitable for a simple partial nephrectomy, and thus best treated by total nephrectomy. If angiography suggests a typical RCC and there is no reason to preserve renal parenchyma, total nephrectomy may be the easiest and safest therapy for the patient (Fig 6–1). In some settings the incidental renal mass can present a formidable surgical challenge, and it may be difficult for the patient to appreciate the significance of the problem in the absence of symptoms (Fig 6–2).

RESULTS

The frequency of RCC cases diagnosed as an incidental finding is increasing. Konnak and Grossman[14] found that 13% of all RCCs in their institution between 1961 and 1973 were found incidentally compared with 38% between 1980 and 1987. Their data also suggested that incidental tumors were lower stage and associated with a better prognosis. The corollary of this would be that as the proportion of cases diagnosed in the incidental setting increases, the total survival of patients with RCC would improve. Thompson and Peek[15] have provided data supporting this concept. The low prevalence of RCC would make specific screening or case finding efforts in the general population with CT or ultrasonography inappropriate on the basis of cost and potential morbidity of further diagnostic studies.

SUMMARY

The incidental renal mass will be seen with increasing frequency, and a logical plan for management is valuable. If the lesion is small and easily amenable to an excisional biopsy with a partial nephrectomy, this would be reasonable. If the lesion is likely to be malignant, large, or not ideally suited for a partial nephrectomy, total nephrectomy is the preferred treatment. A percutaneous preoperative biopsy can provide valuable information, but a sampling and interpretative problems frequently prevent biopsy from solving the dilemma.

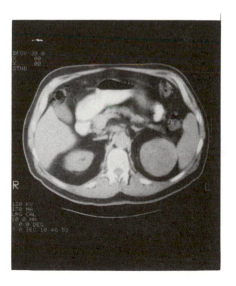 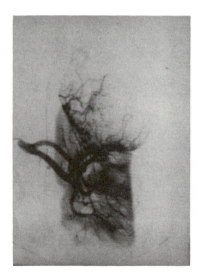

FIG 6–1.
CT scan (*left*) and renal (*right*) angiography by intraarterial digital subtraction angiography on a 75-year-old man with an incidentally discovered renal mass. The lesion is probably malignant, large, and poorly suited for a partial nephrectomy. Radical nephrectomy was performed and RCC confirmed.

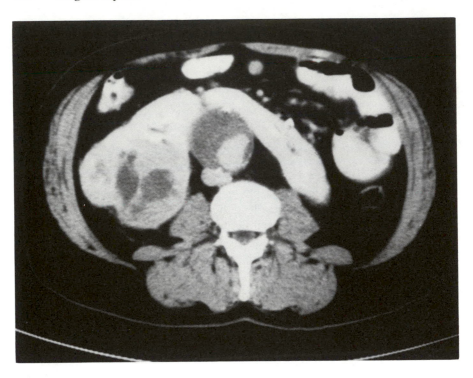

FIG 6–2.
CT scan in a 71-year-old man with an incidentally discovered renal mass in a horseshoe kidney. Also noted was a 6 to 7 cm abdominal aortic aneurysm. Treatment required removal of a portion of the horseshoe kidney and repair of the aneurysm. Pathologic examination confirmed RCC.

REFERENCES

1. Lang EK: Roentgenographic assessment of asymptomatic renal lesions. An analysis of the confidence level of diagnoses established by sequential roentgenographic investigation. *Diagn Radiol* 1973; 109:257–269.
2. Livingston MWD, Jr, Collins TL, Novicki DE: Incidental renal mass. *Urology* 1981; 27:257–259.
3. Zabbo A, Montie JE: Intraoperative consultation for the kidney. *Urol Clin* 1985; 12:405–410.
4. Tada S, Yamagishi J, Kobayashi H, et al: The incidence of simple renal cyst by computed tomography. *Clin Radiol* 1983; 34:437–439.
5. Dalton D, Neiman H, Grayhack JT: The natural history of simple renal cysts: A preliminary study. *J Urol* 1986; 135:905–908.
6. Mostofi FK, Davis CJ, Jr: Tumors and tumor-like lesions of the kidney, *Curr Probl Cancer* 1986; 10:53–114.
7. Bennington JL: Renal adenoma. *World J Urol* 1987; 5:66–70.
8. Mukamel E, Konichezky M, Engelstein D, et al: Incidental small renal tumors accompanying clinically overt renal cell carcinoma. *J Urol* 1988; 140:22–24.

9. Maatman TJ, Novick AC, Tancinco BF, et al: Renal oncocytoma: A diagnostic and therapeutic dilemma. *J Urol* 1984; 132:878–881.

10. Juul N, Torp-Pedersen S, Gronvall S, et al: Ultrasonically guided fine needle aspiration biopsy of renal masses. *J Urol* 1985; 133:579–581.

11. Kiser GC, Totonchy M, Barry JM: Needle tract seeding after percutaneous renal adenocarcinoma aspiration. *J Urol* 1986; 136:1292–1293.

12. Blackley SK, Ladaga L, Woolfitt RA, et al: Ex situ study of the effectiveness of enucleation in patients with renal cell carcinoma. *J Urol* 1988; 140:6–10.

13. Marshall FF, Taxy JB, Fishman EK, et al: The feasibility of surgical enucleation for renal cell carcinoma. *J Urol* 1986; 135:231–234.

14. Konnak JW, Grossman HB: Renal cell carcinoma as an incidental finding. *J Urol* 1985; 134:1094–1096.

15. Thompson IM, Peek M: Improvement in survival of patients with renal cell carcinoma—The role of the serendipitously detected tumor. *J Urol* 1988; 140:487–490.

Part III

Metastatic Diseases

7

The Problem of Metastases

Ronald M. Bukowski, M.D.

METASTATIC DISEASE IN RENAL CELL CARCINOMA

RCC is an unpredictable tumor with a variable natural history. Extensive local or distant spread is unfortunately a common occurrence in patients with this malignancy. The incidence of metastases at the time of diagnosis in patients with this type of cancer has been estimated to be 25%.[1,2] After diagnosis and curative surgical therapy, the incidence of this complication is somewhat variable but has been reported by various authors[3,4] to be from 30% to 50%. The methods of spread in these instances include both local growth through the surrounding capsule with direct extension into the perinephric fat and surrounding structures and distant spread through lymphatic vessels. This latter mode does not necessarily occur in a stepwise manner, with initial spread to the regional lymph nodes being uncommon.[5] Finally, venous invasion is quite common in these tumors and interestingly does not appear to adversely affect prognosis in all instances.[1] Therefore both synchronous and asynchronous metastases occur in patients with RCC, and because of their incidence, they present a significant problem.

The sites of metastatic disease can be quite varied, with the lungs, lymph nodes, and bone being the most common sites.[2,6] In an autopsy series Bennington and Kradjian[7] reported 55% of patients had pulmonary involvement. Isolated pulmonary involvement can also occur and has been reported in 30% of patients with metastases.[8] Finally, another peculiar feature of this tumor is that metastatic disease can occur at odd sites with regions such as the iris, epididymis, and gallbladder being reported.[9]

Survival is limited after the development of metastatic disease. The behavior of RCC, however, can be unpredictable, with certain subsets of patients having extremely indolent disease despite the lack of any therapy. de Kernion et al[3] reported a cumulative survival for 86 patients with metastatic renal carcinoma to be 26% at 2 years. The 5-year survival was 13% in this series. This group, however, did not include patients with synchronous disease. In a larger study Riches et al[10] reported that the crude survival for 443 patients was 4.4% at 3 years and 2.7% at 5 years. Therefore 5-year survival with metastatic renal cancer is uncommon.

Spontaneous Regression

One of the most notable features of RCC has been the observation that idiopathic or spontaneous regression of metastatic disease can occur. This phenomenon interestingly has been reported for primary renal tumors and for metastatic disease. Hellsten et al[11] reported regression, as demonstrated at histologic examination, in 3.4% of primary tumors. This type of regression was associated with fibrosis in the primary tumor. Most reports, however, have focused on regression of metastatic disease, either after nephrectomy or occurring spontaneously. The overall incidence has been estimated to be approximately 0.8% for patients undergoing nephrectomy and 0.4% for nonsurgical-related phenomena.[12] A recent report by Oliver,[13] in which 69 patients with RCC were observed until symptomatic progression occurred, noted unexplained or spontaneous regression of metastatic lesions in five patients in the group (7%). All patients had bidimensionally measurable disease and histologically proved renal cancer. The regressions were complete in three instances and partial in two, with a duration of 6 to 48 months. The likelihood is that this group was biased, since patients were selected by virtue of lack of symptoms. Therefore the incidence figure reported may represent an overestimate of this phenomenon. These reports, however, demonstrate that with objective criteria, spontaneous tumor regression does occur. The exact causes for this phenomenon remain unclear, but speculation includes host factors such as the immune response as a possible cause.

Surgical Therapy for Metastatic Renal Cell Carcinoma

Because idiopathic regression of metastases is a rare phenomenon in these patients, multiple therapeutic interventions have been explored. Historically, RCC has been thought to be unresponsive to conventional therapeutic modalities such as chemotherapy, therefore surgery has assumed a prominent role in dealing with metastatic disease. In the subset of patients who either at the time of presentation or at a later date develop a solitary metastasis, surgical removal can result in prolonged survival. This concept was recognized at the turn of the century by Scudder.[14] Since then, numerous reports[15, 16] have been published in which solitary metastases occurring in most any organ of the body have been noted. The overall incidence of this phenomenon is uncertain but has been estimated to range from 2% to 4%.[16, 17] Surgical resection of these metastases has been recommended, and 5-year survival in this group of patients has been estimated to be 30% to 35%.[18] Recently, the possibility that removal of multiple pulmonary metastases may also be beneficial has been raised, and surgical approaches employing this technique are now being investigated.

In the group of patients who initially have metastatic disease and the primary tumor in place, adjunctive nephrectomy has been advocated because of the possibility of spontaneous regression of metastases. This has been combined with embolic infarction, hormonal therapy, or immunotherapy. In a critical review of this phenomenon,[19] improved survival for a group with only bone metastases was noted when compared with patients with metastases in other sites. The estimate of spontaneous regression of metastatic disease occurring in patients after adjunctive nephrectomy in this report[19] was noted to be 0.8% (review of 474 patients). Thus although spontaneous regressions can occur, they are distinctly uncommon in this setting, and the use of adjunctive nephrectomy should be reserved for patients with minimal metastatic disease or for those having osseous metastases alone.

Systemic Therapy for Metastatic Renal Cell Carcinoma

Because of the frequency of metastatic disease in patients with RCC, systemic therapy of various types has been intensively studied. In view of the unpredictable behavior of this tumor and evidence suggesting that host factors may be capable of modifying the course of the disease (spontaneous regressions), various attempts to augment the immune response in these patients have been made. Additionally, the use of cytotoxic and/or hormonal agents also has received attention as a possible therapy.

Chemotherapy.—Multiple antineoplastic agents have been used as treatment for metastatic RCC. Recent reviews[20, 21] of this subject have noted the overall response rate to all agents to be disappointingly small. All classes of drugs have received trials in this disease including newer agents such as the epipodophyllotoxins,[22] cisplatin,[23] and the anthracycline antibiotics.[24] Dose intensification has also been examined, and in preliminary studies[25] with autologous bone marrow transplantation followed by high dose chemotherapy, no improvement in response rates was seen. A recent report[26] has examined the concept of continuous infusion of floxuridine (5-FUDR), an antimetabolite that was given by means of a programmable constant infusion pump with most medication administered at approximately 6:00 PM. The authors[26] reported that toxicity was minimal and that in 18 patients who could be evaluated, 6 responses were observed. This concept of programmable drug delivery with 5-FUDR is now being examined in a more detailed and critical fashion. Chemotherapy, however, remains of minimal use for patients with metastatic renal carcinoma and is considered investigational.

Hormonal Therapy.—The rationale for the use of hormonal therapy in patients with metastatic RCC is based on encouraging results obtained in various animal models of renal cancer in the 1940s. It was demonstrated that these tumors could be suppressed with hormonal agents such as medroxyprogesterone acetate (Provera)[27] and testosterone.[28] The topic was reviewed by Bloom,[29] who reported a series of patients in whom the objective tumor response rate was 7% to 25%, with the overall regression rate at 16%. Multiple studies with progesterone derivatives,[30] androgens,[20] estrogen antagonists,[31] and hormonal agents combined with chemotherapy[20, 32] were then performed. Hrushesky and Murphy[33] reviewed the recent trials and reported that the overall response rate with all types of hormonal manipulation is less than 2%. Currently it appears that hormonal therapy rarely produces objective tumor regression in these patients and that if responses are seen, they are generally incomplete, with no survival benefit for patients.

Another approach with hormonal therapy is to administer it in combination with another modality. Depo-Provera was recently used in combination with angioinfarction followed by adjunctive nephrectomy in patients with metastatic RCC. This was based on an observation by Almgard et al,[34] who noted that in certain patients undergoing embolic occlusion of the renal circulation followed by nephrectomy, metastases remained stable for a prolonged period. Swanson et al[35] then investigated this therapy in a prospective manner. They reported a response rate of 24% with this combined modality approach and hypothesized that one possible response mechanism was stimulation of the patients' immune response as a result of the release of tumor antigen into the circulation. Attempts to reproduce the results seen in this study by the Southwest Oncology Group[36] were unsuccessful.

Biologic Response Modifiers

Because of the resistance of RCC to standard therapies such as chemotherapy and hormonal therapy and because of the speculation that the spontaneous regression may represent immunologic rejection of a tumor, attempts to use biologic approaches as treatment for this neoplasm have been advocated. Initial trials in the 1970s utilized poorly characterized agents such as bacillus Calmette-Guérin[37] or transfer factor.[38] Responses were noted, and this provided a rationale for more detailed studies.

In the 1970s it was recognized that bacillus Calmette-Guérin may augment the immune response in a nonspecific fashion. Morales and Eidinger[37] described 10 patients with renal carcinoma who received intradermal bacillus Calmette-Guérin. Four of these patients developed partial responses. Attempts to reproduce this, however, have failed.[39] Two other approaches, one utilizing immune ribonucleic acid (RNA)[40] and the second using transfer factor,[38] were also investigated at approximately the same time. Immune RNA was composed of RNA-rich extracts prepared from xenogeneic tissue removed from animals immunized with renal cancer. Transfer factor was prepared from peripheral blood mononuclear cells obtained from normal donors; these cells had the ability to transfer immune information such as delayed hypersensitivity.[38] In both these instances isolated responses in patients with metastatic renal cancer were seen but were infrequent. Because these agents were poorly characterized and mechanisms of actions uncertain, investigations with these types of BRMs have been largely abandoned.

Attempts to enhance the immune response in patients by immunization with tumor cells or tumor antigen (active specific immunotherapy) have also been made. Animal experiments[41] demonstrated that immunization with tumor cells and an adjuvant such as bacillus Calmette-Guérin prevented tumor growth. Tumor cell suspensions that were radiated and mixed with adjuvants such as bacillus Calmette-Guérin or Corynebacterium parvum[42] were then utilized in patients with renal cancer. Again tumor regressions occurred, but they continued to be infrequent. Extracts of tumor cell membranes that were polymerized were then used as immunizing agents by Tallberg et al[43] and Neidhardt et al.[44] The preparations were thought to contain tumor-associated antigens. The latter study[44] was followed by a randomized trial[45] in which patients received either active specific immunotherapy or Depo-Provera. Three responses in the patients receiving the active specific immunotherapy and none in those receiving progesterone were reported. Interestingly, the patients who received immunologic therapy also had slightly longer survival times and delayed disease progression. Presently, one must conclude that active specific immunization in this disease has minimal effects but that regressions do occur. As with other modalities, the responses are infrequent and generally brief.

The recognition that interferon may possibly augment host immune responses provided a rationale for trials utilizing these agents in patients with renal cancer. Because of the recognized responses of renal cancer to other forms of immune therapy, interferon therefore was investigated. Early studies were performed with partially purified leukocyte interferon obtained from human peripheral blood leukocytes. In an early publication Quesada et al[46] reported partial regression of metastatic renal cancer in five of 19 patients. All patients who responded had lymph node or lung metastases. In subsequent studies[47] with a similar interferon preparation partial tumor regressions were again observed, but they were less frequent. The mechanism of action of interferon in these studies remains unknown. Whether it was mediating a direct antiproliferative effect or whether the effects were by means of host immune effector mechanisms is unclear. Recombinant α-interferon (rHuIFNα2A, rHuIFNα2B) became available in the 1980s after successful isolation of the coding for DNA for α-interferon. Large scale production took place, and trials utilizing various schedules and dose levels of the recombinant products have been performed.[48,49] These studies continue to demonstrate that tumor regressions occur with the recombinant interferons but that they are generally partial. Recently the overall response rate to α-interferons (both natural and recombinant) has been estimated to be 14% in over 400 patients.[50] These responses are generally partial and occur predominately in patients with lung metastases in whom primary tumors have been removed. Because of this consistent activity, the use of interferon in an adjuvant setting where the primary tumor has been removed but where there is a significant chance of relapse is now being investigated.

Several other interferon species have also been produced by recombinant DNA techniques, including β- and γ-interferons. These preparations have been utilized in patients with metastatic renal cancer,[51, 52] and again tumor regressions were noted. It appears that the interferons as a class of agents can mediate tumor regression in these patients, but the frequency of response is still low and approximately 10% to 15% for all preparations.

The description of the T cell growth factor called interleukin 2 (IL-2) in the 1970s[53] and its subsequent production with recombinant DNA technology[54] were followed by a studies utilizing this agent alone or in combination with adoptive immunotherapy in patients with renal cancer. The activities of IL-2 are multiple, but specifically it appears to augment the cytolytic activity of natural killer cells and cytotoxic T cells and to induce a differentiation and growth of various T cells.[55] The availability of this T cell growth factor has made possible the development of adoptive immunotherapy regimens.[56] Peripheral blood lymphocytes proliferate when cultured with IL-2, become cytotoxic to fresh tumor cells (lymphokine-activated killer cells), and then can be collected and reinfused into patients. Investigations with IL-2 alone or in combination with lymphokine-activated cells in patients with metastatic renal carcinoma are now in progress.

IL-2 alone has been used in various doses and schedules,[56, 57] and it is now recognized that patients can demonstrate tumor regressions and that these may be complete in selected patients. Like previous BRM trials, soft-tissue and pulmonary metastases are the most frequent to respond, but additionally bone metastases have also been reported to respond. Some of the responses reported have been complete, seem quite durable, and therefore may represent a therapeutic advance. Figures 7–1 and 7–2 demonstrate a complete response to high dose rIL-2 in a patient with metastatic renal cancer and pleural-based metastases. The response duration in this instance is now greater than 8 months. The toxicity of high dose IL-2 is significant, however, and includes fever, chills, anemia, weight gain, and nausea.[56] Additionally, hypotension requiring pressor agents and respiratory distress requiring intubation have been reported. Because IL-2 given as a bolus in high doses has significant toxicity, different schedules such as continuous infusion have been developed.[58] Toxicity appears less but is dose related. More important, responses have been seen. The overall response rate to IL-2 alone is still unclear, and further investigations of continuous infusion regimens and high dose schedules are needed.

Finally, immunomodulatory chemotherapy such as low dose cyclophosphamide (300 mg/m²) has been combined with IL-2.[59] This type of approach was designed to reduce the immunosuppression associated with malignancy and possibly increase the efficacy of IL-2. Results are preliminary, but objective tumor regressions in patients with malignancy receiving this type of treatment have been reported.[59]

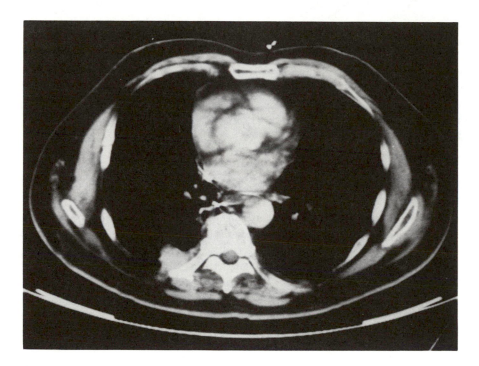

FIG 7–1.
CT scan of chest demonstrates right-sided pleural-based metastasis in patient with metastatic renal carcinoma.

Recently, combined cytokine therapy has also been investigated in both preclinical models and in patients. Synergism in preclinical murine tumor models with IL-2 and rHuIFNαA/D[60] has been reported. Phases I and II trials of the combination of rIL-2 and rHuIFNα2A have therefore been initiated. Preliminary reports[61] in patients with renal cancer demonstrate responses, but the frequency of response, best schedule, and mechanism of the synergism are still uncertain. Some of the observed responses have been interesting, and in Figures 7–3 to 7–6 the chest x-ray films of a patient with synchronous metastatic disease and the primary tumor in place, who had hypercalcemia and erythrocytosis, illustrate almost complete regression of pulmonary metastases in this patient after therapy with rIL2 and rHuIFNα2A.

The application of adoptive immunotherapy to various human malignancies has been made possible by the availability of recombinant IL-2, and preclinical findings indicating administration of lymphokine-activated killer cells and IL-2 in murine tumor models[62] may have significant antitumor effects. Rosenberg et al[56] and West et al[63] have studied this treatment approach in patients and reported over 40 patients with metastatic renal cancer who received IL-2 and lymphokine-activated killer cells.

The methods of IL-2 administration differed, but responses were seen. Complete responses were noted and may be more frequent when compared with IL-2 alone, with the overall response rate at over 20%.[56, 63] With this approach it appears that response frequency may be slightly higher when compared with other methods, but this observation is preliminary, and further studies in this area are needed. Toxicity with these regimens, however, is significant and certainly more substantial when compared with agents such as interferon. This limits the potential application of this type of treatment, and attempts to modify the side effects by employing different schedules and doses of IL-2 are now underway.

The recognition in animal models[64] that lymphocytes obtained from the tumor (tumor-infiltrating lymphocytes) may be more effective when used for adoptive immunotherapy than are peripheral blood lymphocytes has now prompted investigators[65] to utilize this population of cells for treatment. It has been demonstrated[66] that most lymphocytes in primary renal tumors and metastatic tumors are T cells and that these can be readily grown and expanded in vitro with IL-2. Techniques for large scale cultures have been developed, and preliminary studies utilizing tumor-infiltrating lymphocytes with and without IL-2 are now underway. The potential efficacy of this form of adoptive immunotherapy in patients with renal carcinoma remains unclear but theoretically appears to represent an improvement.

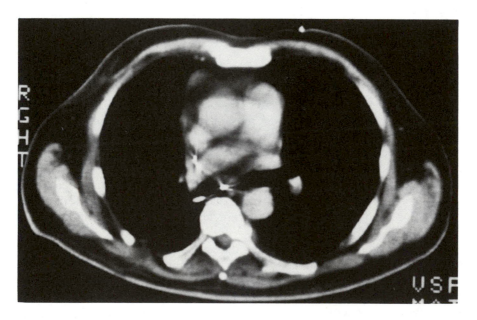

FIG 7–2.
CT scan of chest of patient in Figure 7–1 demonstrates complete resolution of metastatic lesion after IL-2 therapy.

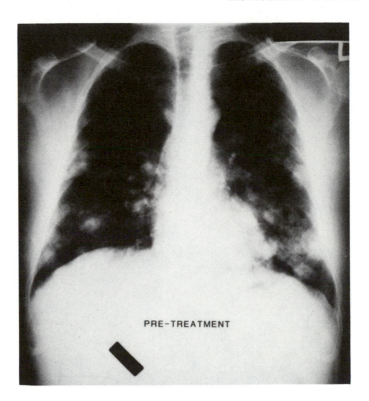

PRE-TREATMENT

FIG 7–3.
Chest x-ray film of patient with metastatic RCC demonstrates multiple pulmonary metastases.

Finally, the availability of other growth factors such as the hematopoietic growth factor GM-CSF and IL-1 will allow their efficacy as potential BRMs in patients with RCC to be examined.

The use of monoclonal antibodies in patients with malignancies has allowed substantial advances in our attempts to understand tumor antigens and characterize malignant cells. The work in RCC[67] has demonstrated that most renal carcinomas have tumor-associated antigens that appear to identify them as proximal tubular cells and that they likely arise from this area. Attempts to utilize monoclonal antibodies as therapeutic agents have been made over the past 5 years. Two groups[67, 68] have reported trials of conjugated and unconjugated antibodies in patients with renal cancer, with an occasional response seen. Generally the toxicity has been moderate; however, therapeutic efficacy has been minimal. Recently, studies employing conjugated antibodies (e.g., radioimmunoconjugates) have been undertaken in attempts to improve efficacy. These studies are underway and may provide information concerning the utility of this treatment approach for patients with renal tumors.

In conclusion, systemic approaches to the treatment of RCC remain poor, but recent developments are interesting and may provide clues to more efficient methods of management of this tumor utilizing immunologic techniques. From the available data it does appear that renal cancer may regress when treated with various BRMs. The responses remain infrequent, but findings of complete tumor regressions in patients receiving IL-2 with or without lymphkine-activating killer cells that appear durable may be of significance. These approaches remain investigational, but within the next several years may provide the basis for more successful management of advanced and/or metastatic RCC.

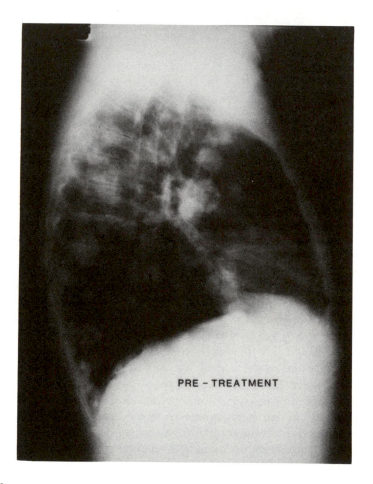

PRE – TREATMENT

FIG 7–4.
Chest x-ray film of patient with metastatic RCC demonstrates multiple pulmonary metastases.

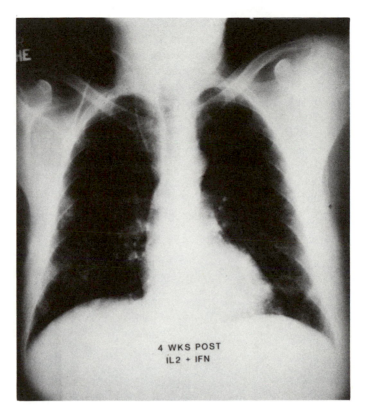

FIG 7–5.
Chest x-ray film of patient in Figures 7–3 and 7–4 demonstrates near total resolution of pulmonary metastases after 4 weeks of therapy with rIL-2 and rHuIFNα2A.

Palliative Therapy for Metastatic Renal Cell Carcinoma

New systemic approaches to therapy in patients with RCC are available, but most patients with metastatic disease still do not benefit from these treatments. In view of the varied sites affected by tumor spread, attempts at palliation generally differ depending on the area affected or symptoms produced.

In patients with synchronous metastatic disease, and in whom the primary tumor has not been removed, alleviation of symptoms referable to the local tumor (e.g., pain or hematuria) has been used as an argument for palliative nephrectomy. Analysis of these patients, however, suggests that symptoms requiring surgery seldom develop, and other means of alleviating symptoms occasionally produced by these tumors may be preferable. Fever can be controlled by indomethacin, 25 mg four times a day, and/or by use of systemic corticosteroids. Hematuria and pain produced by the primary lesion can be alleviated by percutaneous renal artery occlusion.[69] The rarity of tumor regression as noted previously does not justify nephrectomy in this setting.

The systemic effects of RCC may be related to either the primary tumor or the effects of metastases. Fever occurs in 16% of patients with renal tumors,[70] and its presence does not necessarily correlate with tumor size, presence of necrosis, or spread. Use of antiinflammatory agents such as indomethacin or corticosteroids can aid in control of this symptom. Hypercalcemia in patients with RCC can result from production of a parahormone-like material by the primary tumor[70] or skeletal metastases. Use of agents such as mithramycin, 25 μg/kg intravenously, or sodium didronate can effectively control this problem.

Osseous metastases are the second most common type in these patients, and therefore palliation of the symptoms produced by this complication has an important role in management. Radiation therapy is generally used for control of bone pain, and response in terms of alleviation of symptoms occurs in over 75% of patients.[71] No relation between the doses given and the response has

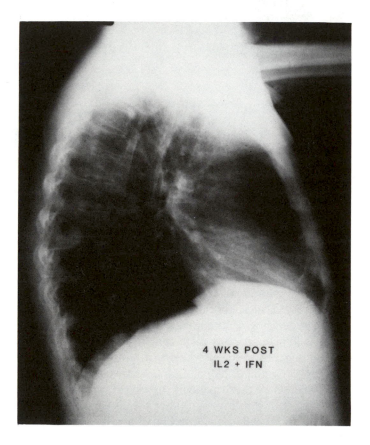

FIG 7–6.
Chest x-ray film of patient in Figures 7–3 and 7–4 demonstrates near total resolution of pulmonary metastases after 4 weeks of therapy with rIL-2 and rHuIFNα2A.

been noted, however. In areas of weight bearing, surgical approaches (e.g., total hip replacement) may be useful. In the subset of patients with disease in the bone only, judicious application of these procedures can yield significant palliation.

Finally, neurologic symptoms caused by brain and/or spinal cord metastases can develop. The standard of therapy involves use of irradiation and steroids (e.g., dexamethasone [Decadron]). A review of this area,[71] however, notes that a measurable response in the central nervous system is uncommon and palliation poor. This is likely related to the limited tolerance of central nervous system tissue to radiation, limiting the dose administered. When surgical approaches are not indicated or possible, this method remains the best choice for treatment. In conclusion, when investigational treatment approaches for metastatic RCC are not possible or indicated, significant palliation may be possible with traditional methods of symptom control, radiation therapy, and occasionally surgery.

REFERENCES

1. Skinner DG, Calvin RB, Vermillion CD, et al: Diagnosis and management of renal cell carcinoma. A clinical and pathologic study of 309 cases. *Cancer* 1971; 28:1165–1177.
2. Ritchie AWS, Chisholm GD: The natural history of renal carcinoma. *Semin Oncol* 1983; 10:390–400.
3. DeKernion JB, Rammings KD, Smith RB: The natural history of metastatic renal cell carcinoma: A computer analysis. *J Urol* 1978; 128:148–152.
4. Rafla S: Renal cell carcinoma: Natural history and results of treatment. *Cancer* 1970; 25:26–32.
5. Hellsten S, Berge T, Linell E: Clinically unrecognized renal carcinoma: Aspects of tumor morphology, lymphatic and hematogenous metastatic spread. *Br J Urol* 1983; 55:166–170.
6. Patel NP, Lavengood RW: Renal cell carcinoma: Natural history and results of treatment. *J Urol* 1978; 119:722–726.
7. Bennington JL, Kradjian RM: Distribution of metastases from renal carcinoma, in Bennington JL, Kradjian RM (eds): *Renal Carcinoma.* Philadelphia, WB Saunders Co, 1967.
8. Kutty K, Varkey B: Incidence and distribution of intrathoracic metastases from renal cell carcinoma. *Arch Intern Med* 1984; 144:273–276.
9. Tabara WS, Mchio AM, Aftimos GP: Metastatic renal cell adenocarcinoma: Renal tumors. *Proceedings of the First International Symposium on Kidney Tumors.* New York, Liss, 1982, pp 317–336.
10. Riches E: The natural history of renal tumors, in: *Tumors of the Kidney and Ureter.* Edinburgh, United Kingdom, Churchill Livingstone, 1984, pp 124–134.
11. Hellsten S, Berge T, Wehlin L: Unrecognized renal cell carcinoma. Clinical and pathologic aspects. *Scand J Urol Nephrol* 1981; 8:273–278.
12. McCune CS: Immunologic therapies of kidney carcinoma. *Semin Oncol* 1983; 10:431–436.

13. Oliver RTD: Unexplained "spontaneous" regression and its relevance to the clinical behaviour of renal cell carcinoma and its response to interferon. *Proc Am Soc Clin Oncol* 1987; 6:98.
14. Scudder CL: The bone metastases of hypernephroma. *Ann Surg* 1906; 44:851–865.
15. Barney JD, Churchill EJ: Adenocarcinoma of the kidney with metastasis to the lung cured by nephrectomy and lobectomy. *J Urol* 1939; 42:269–276.
16. Tobia BM, Whitmore WF: Solitary metastasis from renal cell carcinoma. *J Urol* 1975; 114:836–838.
17. O'Dea MJ, Zincke H, Utz DC, et al: The treatment of renal cell carcinoma with solitary metastasis. *J Urol* 1978; 120:540–542.
18. Kjaer M, Engelholm SA: The clinical course and prognosis of patients with renal adenocarcinoma with solitary metastasis. *Int J Radiat Oncol Biol Phys* 1982; 8:1691–1698.
19. Montie JE, Stewart BH, Straffon RA, et al: The role of adjunctive nephrectomy in patients with metastatic renal cell carcinoma. *J Urol* 1977; 117:272–275.
20. Poster DS, Bruno S, Penta JS, et al: Current status of chemotherapy, hormonal therapy, and immunotherapy in the treatment of renal cell carcinoma. *Am J Clin Oncol* 1982; 5:53–60.
21. Luderer RC, Opipari MI, Perrotta AL: Treatment of metastatic renal cell carcinoma: Review of experience and world literature. *J Am Oncol Assoc* 1978; 77:590–603.
22. Hire EA, Samson MK, Fraile RJ, et al: Use of VM-26 as a single agent in the treatment of renal carcinoma. *Cancer Clin Trials* 1979; 2:293–295.
23. Rossof AH, Talley RW, Stephens R, et al: Phase II evaluation of cis-Dichlorodiamminoplatinum (II) in advanced malignancies of the genitourinary and gynecologic organs: A Southwest Oncology Group Study. *Cancer Treat Rep* 1979; 63:1557–1564.
24. O'Bryan RM, Luce JK, Talley RW: Phase II evaluation of adriamycin in human neoplasia. *Cancer* 1973; 32:1–8.
25. Phillips GL, Fay JW, Herzig GP, et al: Intensive 1,3-bis(2-chlorethyl)-1-nitrosourea (BCNU) NSC 4366650 and cryopreserved autologous marrow transplantation for refractory cancer. *Cancer* 1983; 52:1792–1802.
26. Hrushesky WJM, Roemeling R, Rabatin J, et al: Continuous FUDR infusion is effective in progressive renal cell cancer (RCC). *Proc Am Soc Clin Oncol* 1987; 6:108.
27. Bloom HJG, Dukes CE, Mitchley BCV: The estrogen-induced renal tumor of the Syrian hamster. Hormone treatment and possible relationship to carcinoma of the kidney in man. *Br J Cancer* 1963; 17:611.
28. Harris DT: Hormonal therapy and chemotherapy of renal cell carcinoma. *Semin Oncol* 1983; 10:422–430.
29. Bloom HJG: Medroxyprogesterone acetate (Provera) in treatment of metastatic renal cancer. *Br J Cancer* 1971; 25:250–261.
30. Stolbach LL, Begg CB, Hall T, et al: Treatment of renal carcinoma: A phase III randomized trial of oral medroxyprogesterone (Provera), hydroxyurea, and nafoxidine. *Cancer Treat Rep* 1981; 65:689–692.
31. Weiselberg L, Budman D, Vinciguerra V, et al: Tamoxifen in uresectable hypernephroma: A phase II trial and review of the literature. *Cancer Clin Trials* 1981; 4:195–198.
32. Bell DR, Araney RS, Fischer RJ, et al: High dose methotrexate with leucovorin rescue, vinblastine, and bleomycin with or without tamoxifen in metastatic renal cell carcinoma. *Cancer Treat Rep* 1984; 68:587–590.
33. Hrushesky WJ, Murphy GP: Current status of the therapy of advanced renal carcinoma. *J Surg Oncol* 1977; 9:277–286.

34. Almgard LE, Fernstrom I, Haverling M, et al: Treatment of renal adenocarcinoma by embolic occlusion of the renal circulation. *Br J Urol* 1973; 45:474–479.
35. Swanson DA, Wallace S, Johnson DE: The role of embolization and nephrectomy in the treatment of metastatic renal carcinoma. *Urol Clin North Am* 1980; 7:719–730.
36. Gottesman JE, Crawford ED, Grossman HB, et al: Infarction—Nephrectomy for metastatic renal carcinoma. A Southwest Oncology Group Study. *Urology* 1985; 25:248–250.
37. Morales A, Eidinger D: Bacillus Calmette-Guerin in the treatment of adenocarcinoma of the kidney. *J Urol* 1976; 115:377–380.
38. Montie JE, Bukowski RM, Deodhar S, et al: Immunotherapy of disseminated renal cell carcinoma with transfer factor. *J Urol* 1977; 177:553–556.
39. Morales A, Wilson JL, Pater JL, et al: Cytoreductive surgery and systemic bacillus Calmette-Guerin therapy in metastatic renal cancer: A phase II trial. *J Urol* 1982; 127:230–235.
40. DeKernion JB, Ramming KP: The therapy of renal adenocarcinoma with immune RNA. *Invest Urol* 1980; 17:378–381.
41. Zbar B, Canti G, Rapp JH, et al: Immunoprophylaxis of syngeneic methylcholanthrene-induced murine sarcomas with bacillus calmette-guerin and tumor cells. *Cancer Res* 1980; 40:1036–1042.
42. McCune CS, Schapira DV, Henshaw EC: Specific immunotherapy of advanced renal carcinoma: Evidence for the polyclonality of metastases. *Cancer* 1981; 47:1984–1987.
43. Tallberg T, Tykka H, Mahlberg K, et al: Active specific immunotherapy with supportive measures in the treatment of palliatively nephrectomized renal adenocarcinoma patients. *Eur Urol* 1985; 11:233–243.
44. Neidhardt JA, Murphy SG, Hennick LA, et al: Active specific immunotherapy of stage IV renal carcinoma with aggregated tumor antigen adjuvant. *Cancer* 1980; 46:1128–1135.
45. Neidhardt JA, Gagen M, Young D, et al: A randomized study of polymerized tumor antigen admixed with adjuvant (PTA) for therapy of renal cancer. *Proc Am Soc Clin Oncol* 1983; 2:49.
46. Quesada Jr, Swanson DA, Trindale A, et al: Renal cell carcinoma: anti-tumor effects of leukocyte interferon. *Cancer Res* 1983; 43:940–945.
47. Kirkwood J, Harris J, Vera R, et al: Randomized trial of low and high leukocyte interferon in metastatic renal cell carcinoma. *Cancer Res* 1985; 45:863–867.
48. Quesada JR, Gutterman JV, Rios A: Investigational therapy of renal cell carcinoma with recombinant alpha interferon. *Proc Am Assoc Cancer Res* 1983; 24:195.
49. Kempf RA, Grunberg SM, Daniels JR, et al: Recombinant interferon α-2 (Intron A) in a phase II study of renal cell carcinoma. *J Biol Response Mod* 1986; 5:27–35.
50. Krown SE: Therapeutic options in renal cell carcinoma. *Semin Oncol* 1985; 4:13–17.
51. Rinehart J, Malspeis L, Young D, et al: Phase I/II trial of human recombinant β-interferon serine in patients with renal cell carcinoma. *Cancer Res* 1986; 46:5364–5367.
52. Rinehart JJ, Young D, Laforge J, et al: Phase I/II trial of recombinant gamma interferon in patients with renal cell carcinoma: immunologic and biologic effects. *J Biol Response Mod* 1987; 6:302–312.
53. Morgan DA, Ruscetti FW, Gallo R: Selective in vitro growth of T lymphocytes from normal human bone marrows. *Science* 1976; 193:1007–1008.
54. Rosenberg SA, Grimm EA, McGrogan M, et al: Biological activity of recombinant human interleukin-2 produced in *Escherichia coli. Science* 1984; 223:1412–1414.

55. Hefeneider SH, Conlon PJ, Henney CS, et al: In vivo interleukin-2 administration augments the generation of alloreactive cytolytic T lymphocytes and resident natural killer cells. *J Immunol* 1983; 130:222–227.

56. Rosenberg SA, Lotze MT, Muul LM, et al: A progress report on the treatment of 157 patients with advanced cancer using lymphokine-activated killer cells and interleukin-2 or high dose interleukin-2 alone. *N Engl J Med* 1987; 316:889–897.

57. Lotze MT, Chang AE, Seipp CA, et al: High-dose recombinant interleukin-2 in the treatment of patients with disseminated cancer: Responses, treatment-related morbidity, and histologic findings. *JAMA* 1986; 256:3117–3124.

58. Thompson JA, Lee DJ, Cox W, et al: Recombinant interleukin-2 toxicity, pharmacokinetics, and immunomodulatory effects in a phase I trial. *Cancer Res* 1987; 47:4202–4207.

59. Mitchell MS, Kempf RA, Harel W, et al: Effectiveness and tolerability of low dose cyclophosphamide and low dose intravenous interleukin-2 in disseminated melanoma. *J Clin Oncol* 1988; 6:409–424.

60. Brunda MJ, Tarnowski D, Davateks K: Interaction of recombinant interferons with recombinant interleukin-2: Differential effects on natural killer cell activity and interleukin-2 activated killer cells. *Int J Cancer* 1986; 37:787–793.

61. Bukowski RM, Osgood B, Sergi J, et al: Phase IA/IB trial of interleukin-2 and interferon-α: Results in metastatic renal cell carcinoma (abstract). *J Urol* 1988; 139:283A.

62. Rosenberg SA, Lotze MT, Mule JJ: New approaches to the immunotherapy of cancer using interleukin 2. *Ann Intern Med* 1988; 108:853–864.

63. West WH, Taver KW, Yannelli JR, et al: Constant-infusion recombinant interleukin-2 in adoptive immunotherapy of advanced cancer. *N Engl J Med* 1987; 316:898–905.

64. Rosenberg SA, Spiess P, Lafreniere R: A new approach to the adoptive immunotherapy of cancer with tumor-infiltrating lymphocytes. *Science* 1986; 223:1318–1321.

65. Topalian SL, Solomon D, Avis FP, et al: Immunotherapy of patients with advanced cancer using tumor-infiltrating lymphocytes and recombinant interleukin-2: A pilot study. *J Clin Oncol* 1988; 6:839–853.

66. Finke J, Tubbs R, Connelly B, et al: Tumor infiltrating lymphocytes in patients with renal cell carcinoma: Response to IL2 (abstract). *J Urol* 1988; 139:283A.

67. Bander NH: Monoclonal antibodies in urologic oncology. *Cancer* 1987; 60:658–667.

68. Lange P, Vessella RL, Chiou RK, et al: Monoclonal antibodies in human renal cell carcinoma and their use in radioimmune localization and therapy of tumor xenograft. *Surgery* 1985; 98:143–150.

69. Bracken RB, Johnson DE, Goldstein HM, et al: Percutaneous transfemoral renal artery occlusion in patients with renal carcinoma. *Urology* 1975; 6:6–10.

70. Cronin RE, Kaehny WD, Miller PD, et al: Renal cell carcinoma: Unusual systemic manifestations. *Medicine* 1976; 55:291–311.

71. Halperin EC, Harisiadis L: The role of radiation therapy in the management of metastatic renal cell carcinoma. *Cancer* 1983; 51:614–617.

Index